SWIMMING
a lifelong activity

SWIMMING

a lifelong activity

JOHN LOVESEY

WITH TRAINING SCHEDULES
BY HAMILTON SMITH
Director of British Swimming Coaches Association

WORLD'S WORK LTD
PUBLISHED IN CONJUNCTION WITH
THE SUNDAY TIMES

Series edited by
John Lovesey
Sports Editor, *The Sunday Times*

JOGGING
for fitness and pleasure
Cliff Temple

ORIENTEERING
Norman Harris

EVERYWOMAN
her guide to fitness
Chris Oram

FITNESS AFLOAT
sculling rowing, and canoeing
Richard Burnell

FITNESS ON FOOT
climbing and walking for pleasure
Peter Gillman

CYCLING
fitness on wheels
John Wilcockson

Text copyright © by John Lovesey 1978
Training schedules copyright © by Hamilton Smith 1978
Inside photographs copyright © by Chris Smith 1978
Drawings of swimming strokes copyright © by
John Grimwade 1978
Heart drawings copyright © by Sidney Woods 1978
All rights reserved
Published in Great Britain by World's Work Ltd
The Windmill Press, Kingswood, Tadworth, Surrey
In conjunction with *The Sunday Times*
Printed in Great Britain by
Richard Clay (The Chaucer Press) Ltd, Bungay, Suffolk
SBN 437 09050 7

Contents

Foreword

This book is written primarily for the adult who can swim, who feels the need to get fit and needs a small push. But it might apply to anybody of any age who has not regularly exercised. I have attempted to explain why it is important to keep fit and, assuming the reader is convinced, training schedules by Hamilton Smith have been included to help in attaining this objective. Although this is not an instructional book in the conventional sense, helpful illustrations of the four competitive strokes have been included. Two easy, non-competitive strokes are also described in sufficient detail for the less-competent swimmer to be able to increase his repertoire, and thereby pleasure and progress.

It needs only to be emphasised to anybody who has not been exercising that they should begin gently and steadily. It can be dangerous to attempt too much too soon. Swimming is, nevertheless, an extremely safe sport; only remember that you can drown if you swim out of the sight and reach of other people. It is an activity that can be enjoyed by babies before they can even stand and old people who can barely walk. Swimming is enjoyed by the limbless. It is beneficial to people who are injured in many ways.

In years of swimming myself I have never come across a child who did not love the water, if encouraged into it correctly, and I hope this book might persuade people to discover again such innocent pleasure. Swimming can last you a lifetime.

JOHN LOVESEY
May 1978

CHAPTER ONE

Back to the Water

The woman on the front cover of this book is not a model, nor is she an exceptional swimmer. But she exudes a feeling of good health and an enjoyment of living. Until two years ago, however, she suffered constant colds and other taxing illnesses that make so many people's lives miserable. Then she took up regular swimming . . . and blossomed.

Mrs. Jean Chipperfield is in her late thirties, the mother of three children and stepmother to another five. She has four grandchildren. She runs a busy home with her husband, an ex-motor-cycle racer who is now an engineer, helps him with his growing business and holds down a busy job as a pool attendant and swimming instructor. Dealing with mother-and-baby classes is her forte. She eats what she likes, and has a figure that would flatter many of today's teenagers. As for her vitality as a result of exercise, her husband Ken says: 'She's more energetic now. It's a simple thing, a mental attitude really. If you sit around and wait for death, you're dead before your time.'

When Jean Chipperfield feels sluggish, she dives into the pool and emerges 'all alert'. She has discovered the secret: that physical exercise, rather than making you feel tired, gives you extra energy, enhancing *every* aspect of your life. It improves your awareness of yourself, and your appreciation of everything you see and do.

Many men and women have learned this valuable lesson by what I call going back to the water. It is as simple as that. Yet so many people have hardly an inkling of the benefits of swimming. They have grown up either never knowing, or having forgotten, the bounty of a body that is fit as a result of exercise in the water.

What is it about exercise that makes people smile? What

is it about lack of exercise that makes people frown? Observe, for example, the generally expressionless faces behind the steering wheels of cars caught in a rush-hour queue. When they do display an emotion, it is usually because tempers fray. There is no more apt comment on the physical state of human beings today than the unfit driver haranguing a fellow road-user for some minor or imagined misdemeanour.

Threats are uttered, yet the chances are that the man making the threats is not physically up to putting his muscle where his mouth is. He goes red in the face, his muscles are probably slack from lack of use and his respiratory system rotten. If he did make a complete fool of himself and start a fight, he would as like as not collapse with exhaustion, if not high blood pressure or a heart attack.

A well-exercised person is likely to be generally more calm and in control of himself, and unlikely ever to get caught up in such a situation.

In recent years, nothing has brought home to me the need to exercise more than the number of my neighbours, friends, fellow professional men in their forties and fifties who have suffered, often fatally, from some form of coronary heart disease. Sometimes, it seems hardly a month goes by without my hearing that so-and-so round the corner, or across the road, or in the office, has been rushed to a hospital's intensive care unit. Sometimes too late.

It is as if a plague has been visited upon us, bringing bereaved families in its wake. And it is, of course, a modern plague.

We all have to die one day, but why die, if it can be avoided, before our allotted span? It is not a question of being afraid of death; a common, observable characteristic of fit people is that they are less fearful of dying. They at least know that they have had as full and as useful a life as possible. But can anyone die happy knowing that he or she might have had another 20 or 30 years of fully active life if care had been taken? I doubt it.

As a woman, Jean Chipperfield benefits from an advantage her sex has over men, a built-in biological strength that increases her chances of living longer. In particular, a woman's ovarian function appears to give her protection from heart disease. This may occur because nature perhaps arranged matters so that women are enabled to lead more sedentary lives in safety, looking after children and doing the cooking, while men need to be out and about hunting if they are to achieve a normal life expectation. Though this might not appeal to ardent feminists, it fits in with the theory that men can be healthy only while living in accordance with their biological inheritance. It also fits with the fact that though women *do* need to exercise, they do not need to do so much as men to be equally healthy.

What is not in doubt is that truly primitive peoples of the world must have been healthier than most of today's world. The famine, disease and incredibly short life span now found almost universally in the developing countries were never common features of primitive life. 'The advent of civilisation,' agrees one professor of medicine, 'dealt a blow to man's health from which he is only now recovering.'

In developed countries what many women do not realise is that they are *not* recovering. Protected against coronary heart disease before the menopause, they too become susceptible to its ravages afterwards. Female mortality from coronary heart disease is steadily catching up with the male figures. The reason is clear. Women generally stay active longer than men. They still do more cooking and cleaning and they still will walk to the shops into their sixties and seventies and beyond. Modern life has, however, begun to chip away at this activity, with labour-saving devices and car-drives instead of walks.

Women's experience, therefore, illuminates the problem for everybody. They hold the secret to happier and healthier lives, though they themselves are in danger of losing it. Realising this, women could become the frontline force against coronary heart disease. I remember a book appearing, the jokey import of which was that it was a primer for women on how to kill their husbands. It explained that by overfeeding them, you could kill them. The message was thus: *DON'T*. In fact, what women should be doing is not only eating sensibly with their husbands, but exercising also. It will add to life and enjoyment to the years they have together.

It is not meant as a titillating digression here to mention that the actress Leslie Caron once told me in an interview that, like many French people, she believed 'sex is 90 per cent of marriage'. Whether or not you agree with her, there is no question that a great deal of human unhappiness is caused by an unfulfilled sex life. The wife who is too tired, and the husband with an inclination that measures zero, are the stock-in-trade of many a comedian's patter. Such banter makes us laugh because it holds a mirror up to what is all too frequently a fact. What we need to ask ourselves is why an inability to display love for a person close to us is so sadly funny? Is it because we are not physically fit enough to be fulfilled?

It reminds me of a woman swimmer I know in her early sixties, who has the appearance and the body of a woman many years younger, who turned the tables on some people who were chiding her at a party for neither drinking alcohol nor smoking. 'You don't drink and you don't smoke, you can't be much fun,' they said. The lady swimmer replied, impishly: 'You come home with me, and I'll *show* you some fun.'

In this connection, a survey of veteran swimmers in America threw up an impressive statistic in terms of present-day marriage and divorce. Of those who were married, over 70 per cent were still in their first and only marriage. Furthermore, when asked about the level of sexual activity before they began training and at the present time, of the total 258 (150 men and 108 women) who responded, about 1 in 5 said it was higher. The frequency of intercourse ranged from once or twice a week for 106 swimmers; three times for 35; four for 22; five for 14; six for 3; while two reported considerably more activity.

Happiness is an elusive state, and nobody would suggest swimming or any other physical exercise as a panacea for the unsatisfactory way in which we frequently live our lives today. But it will help. There is little doubt of that.

Henry Ford: he unleashed a killer

Remember if you can the moments in your life when you could say that you felt truly happy. It may have been when you received a good examination result, or were given an increase in wages beyond your wildest expectation, or won a race in the school sports. It could also be the day you got married, or when your first child was born. Different events and circumstances make us all more happy or less happy than our fellow human beings. What makes one person laugh may make another cry.

Indeed, the chances are that what we sometimes understand as happiness is really self-gratification. Thus modern men and women may say they feel happy when they move into a new home, buy a new car or spend a small fortune on new clothes. But modern men and women soon discover that such happiness is illusory. So they have to go on searching.

The problem for everybody in the so-called civilised world today is that the illusion is buttressed everywhere. It is shored up in newspaper and colour-supplement advertisements, and in television commercials. Happiness appears to come packaged in deep-pile homes, electronic kitchens and glossy surfaces. Paradise is round the corner in a pub, where virility is poured into pint mugs and romance into saucer-shaped glasses. Heaven is a new car that can accelerate from nought to 90 miles an hour in 60 seconds.

The car is undoubtedly the greatest scourge of our society. When he popularised it, Henry Ford could have had no idea that he was unleashing a killer that would strike down people in middle-age like a medieval plague, for this is what he wrote in an advertisement for the model he put on the market in 1903: 'This car is built for the good of your health to carry you "jarlessly" over any kind of road, to refresh your brain with the luxury of much "outdoorness" and your lungs with the "tonic of tonics" – the

13

right kind of atmosphere.'

Our economic system, it is argued, depends on this projection of the 'good life'. If we do not consume the products of our factories, everybody will suffer. So travelling by car, barely using our arms and legs, has become a way of life. Television has likewise locked us in our living rooms. And alcoholic liquor all too frequently dulls our senses. It is more like a living death.

In sharp contrast to the propaganda we are deluged with by commerce, regular physical recreation gets comparatively little publicity. What happens as a result? A recent social survey found that after leaving school, and by the age of 22, only 27 per cent of men cited physical recreation as their chief leisure activity, only 20 per cent after marriage, and a mere 10 per cent after their first child was born. For women, the percentages were 28, 10 and two respectively.

Watching television is the major leisure activity of the British. It is not just a joke to say that it has replaced sex: the birthrate booms when power strikes are prolonged enough to keep people away from the 'box'.

There are considerable social class differences to be taken into account, and they particularly illustrate the need for education in the leisure area. For example, a study in southern England showed that semi-skilled and unskilled workers took the least exercise, skilled workers rather more, professional men most. In turn, the ultimate effect of this could be read into a recent report on occupation mortality by England's Registrar-General, which showed that in 1970–72, while one-third of all unskilled workers died before retirement age, just over three-quarters of professional men lived to collect their pensions. Death rates for unskilled workers are higher from a whole string of diseases – lung cancer, heart and circulatory troubles, accidents, poisonings and violence. Moreover, workers' wives reflect a similar pattern – raised mortality and greater risk of death during pregnancy.

The problem is that personal preventive medicine has had to find most of its motivation outside the political

14

arena. The amount of time and attention politicians devote to the subject are mere drops in the ocean of their major preoccupations, even if they do understand why it should be of importance. Instead, the major stimulus for more attention to be paid solely to health through physical recreation has come from independent minds outside of political parties, at least in the West.

In a country like East Germany, the position of sport is enshrined in the constitution. Good bodily health there is an embellishment of their social system, the end product of which is the performance of East German sportsmen and women in the Olympics. In the West, the individually-motivated movement may be more significant in the end, its ideology encapsulated in the remark of an American commentator on a mass of marathon runners. He told his listeners that they were not watching a race, they were watching 'philosophy in action'.

What has given birth to this philosophy in action is simply the realisation that whatever possessions one has – detached house, colour television, smart car – nothing is so valuable as good health. Those among us who are middle-aged or older can probably remember that our own parents or grandparents told us that. They knew the truth before it became swamped by advertising. They perceived that happiness can never be total, but that a sense of well-being need not be a passing phase.

Ironically, a more 'liberal' approach within physical education, now rapidly reassessing itself, has not helped. The freedom to choose in schools has meant we have produced a younger generation who may have dabbled in everything from golf to rugby to sailing, or have been so dazzled by choice that they did little physical training at school, and were not really told of the importance of good health throughout life. Thus, when a great deal of discipline flew out of the window, a whole host of problems piled in through the door.

One of the interesting common denominators among men who did basic military training, in the Second World War or later as national servicemen, is the memory of having felt thoroughly fit at least once in their lives. They may not have been fit by the standards of Olympic athletes, but they were drilled, plunged into physical exercise, chivvied over assault courses and at the end felt on top of the world. The physical euphoria they felt then was similar to that experienced after a particularly energetic holiday. Nobody can maintain that feeling all the time, but it is possible, with some personal discipline, to achieve a general fitness that provides valuable rewards.

CHAPTER TWO

The Alligator that Drowned

Is there, I wonder, a cautionary tale in the research work carried out at the Jefferson Medical College in Philadelphia, where two sets of rats were given transplanted cancer? One set was kept inactive in cages, while the others were put on a ferocious regimen of exercise. The keep-fit rats showed considerable resistance to the cancer growth, and in some cases the cancer seemed to disappear completely. The indolent rats were found to have cancers seven times heavier than those who were forced to exercise vigorously.

Nobody, as far as I know, would claim that exercise cures or prevents cancer. It is merely another piece of evidence to put in the balance on the side of physical recreation.

The three major influences in my own life in relation to physical fitness were school, the Services and, most importantly, my parents. I should say immediately that my qualifications for writing this book are not as a swimming coach or competitor. I have competed only on the most casual basis in a swimming pool since leaving school, but the physical and mental benefits I have gained from swimming are enormous.

Throughout my life I have swum whenever and wherever I can (with one exception which we will come to), and in middle-age swimming helped to work startling physical and mental changes in me. Startling enough totally to convince me of the value of exercise and, moreover, to encourage me to set out here briefly what happened.

My mother and father taught me to swim when I was about four. It is the only significant instruction I have ever had in the activity. Like many swimmers, I have learned the strokes I practise from observation, reading and trial and error. Moreover, I am certain I am still improving, if not in terms of speed then certainly in skill. Sport, like most things in life if you approach them with sufficient modesty, is an area in which you can always learn something. One of the particular attractions of swimming is that as you grow older, practising and polishing your technique can mean that you can often outshine a younger swimmer thrashing away energetically but with less skill.

Dr. James E. Counsilman has coached many American swimming champions, including Mark Spitz. He has always found it curious that so many people resign themselves to what he once called 'a lifetime of hard labour in the water'. Counsilman says they hold to a belief that they simply do not have the natural aptitude to swim well, or are not in good enough condition. Over more than two decades, he has studied the strokes of hundreds of swimmers. They have been of all ages and varying degrees of competence. And Counsilman concludes that efficient swimming seldom comes naturally. To satisfy his curiosity about the relevance of natural ability and learning, he even went underwater to study the swimming techniques of a dozen puppies, a two-year-old alligator and a brood of half-grown ducks, none of which had previously swum a stroke. He reported:

'Although the puppies managed well enough on their first venture in the water, it was obvious that their technique improved in subsequent workouts. Most notably, they began to rely increasingly on their forepaws for propulsion, and to minimise the action of their hind legs, utilising them principally as steering devices. On their first try the ducks tended to list to one side and to swim irregular courses. Although it took the ducks only a few days to become accomplished, there was no doubt that they were learning by the simple process of trial and error. The alligator – the creature one might suspect as being the most naturally endowed – failed completely. On its first attempt, after a few futile movements of its tail and legs, the alligator sank to the bottom of the pool and drowned.'

For most land animals, learning to swim is a relatively simple process. Because of the way their limbs are jointed, most of them have no choice but to make their way through the water by 'dog paddling' as efficiently as possible. By contrast, because of the greater flexibility of our joints, humans are able to swim effectively in a number of ways: on our backs, on our sides, or prone.

'Unfortunately,' said Counsilman, 'even when swimming our most efficient stroke, the front crawl, because of the freedom of action we enjoy we are apt to commit a variety of errors. We are liable, for example, to swing our arms too stiffly during one part of the stroke cycle, and we are equally apt to flex our wrist, elbows, shoulders or knees at the wrong moment and in wasteful ways. To put it simply, since there are many things we can do wrong, we have to work harder than other land creatures to get in the right groove.'

Fortunately, water play these days is a recognised part of child development. In every up-to-date infant or nursery classroom you will find a large tray of water containing an assortment of equipment, including sponges, funnels, bottles and things that float and objects that sink. It is there because it plays a part in vocabulary (squeeze, absorb, soak, drip, sprinkle, etc.) socialisation (it involves sharing) and is fun (like swimming).

Getting rid of allergies

At the last school I went to, the importance of health to a good life was drummed into me by a physical training master of the old type. As he evangelised about exercise and keeping oneself clean, he stood straight but relaxed. Unlike some of today's PE teachers, he would not put up with too much familiarity. His influence, however, was immense. He prepared one for the so-called rigours of National Service, the dreaded drill instructor and the assault course.

I mention him because the truth of all that he had to tell became crystal clear later. On leaving the RAF, I was pitch-forked by fortune into sports journalism. At this point, any man or woman who is experiencing a hectic life full of professional or personal pressures can identify with the problems that began to pile up for me. Luckily, my attention was drawn in good time to what was happening to me by very obvious physical symptoms. Too often, the first sign is a sudden heart attack.

My body's reaction to too many late nights, too much food and booze plus hard work, in what I honestly believed was the proper pursuit of my career, was to break out in allergic rashes. These became worse after I had recovered from an attack of infectious hepatitis. Hepatitis attacks the liver and leaves the victim long after feeling rather weak, more likely to tire quickly. The trouble I sensed as time went on, was almost certainly psychosomatic, related in some way to tension at work. When that increased, then so did my tendency to become allergic. Knowing this did not make the allergy easier to cure in conventional medical terms, that is by treatment with drugs.

On one occasion, while I was travelling overseas, such a bad allergic rash broke out on the back of my neck that by the time I arrived home, after failing to find proper treatment abroad, my shirt collar had to be literally peeled away from the infected surface. An antibiotic cream relieved the rash, but did not get at the cause.

By this time, though I would have denied I was unfit and been offended if I had been told as much, I now know that I was distinctly unfit. I was not even swimming very often – for the only time in my life. I was trapped totally in consideration for business and family responsibility. When I was at least 28 pounds overweight, my daughter joked that I was almost in need of a bra. What's more, I found it difficult to keep calm. I was not sleeping well, either.

Whenever I encountered a particularly difficult patch at work, I would observe the usual telltale signs. A rash would begin to appear somewhere under the skin, in the fold of the arms, round the neck, at the back of the knees. If untreated, the rash would get worse. With it would grow a feeling of general debility.

I was by now a busy editorial executive, dealing not simply with creative problems but ones of administration, handling a large and temperamental staff. To keep my allergic rashes at bay, I swallowed anti-histamine tablets and applied creams to the skin. When the situation got too bad, my doctor would provide a steroid-based ointment, while warning of possible side effects. When I discovered how drowsy anti-histamine tablets made me feel, I got friends to obtain a pill in Germany that counteracts this by incorporating within it a shot of caffeine. Finally, I sought specialist treatment.

A medical consultant diagnosed my problem correctly – tension. But I could not accept his treatment. He pre-scribed tranquillisers. Apart from the fact I felt it was a bad thing for a journalist to be tranquillised, these drugs some-how epitomise for me modern man's failure to cope with social and work pressures. If we need tranquillisers, some-thing must be drastically wrong. Taking them won't un-cover what is at fault.

At this point, I remembered particularly the pleasure I had always experienced while swimming. When very young, I had been well aware of the mental relaxation swimming could provide; you forgot everything else. In a pool, I had observed, problems not only diminished, they frequently solved themselves. Looking down at the bottom of a swimming bath, you appeared to be flying free. The result was that the mind became unfettered. You could even swoop and rise, the only sounds being that of your own breathing, and water dancing past your ears. I decided to take up swimming again, to eat less and drink less, and to lose weight.

There is no question that over-training and over-dieting can make one tired and irritable, the very opposite of what should be the aim. I noticed some traces of this in myself, and certainly it is not necessary to exercise as often as I did, swimming some five or six times a week, usually each morning. I was also perhaps cutting down on my food in-take too drastically.

However, two moments in my first year of vigorous middle-age exercise and battle against allergies made it all worthwhile. Firstly, by the time I had worked up to swim-ming 1,000 yards a day – a good round figure which I liked the sound of – I had lost enough weight for the very daughter who had once told me I almost needed a bra, to remark when she next saw me in swimming trunks: 'You look so *thin*.' And secondly, my own sudden observation in a mirror that I had developed muscles I had not seen for years in myself. (A quick glance in a mirror, by the way, is as good a guide to the shape you are in as any scales.)

Most importantly of all, I had found a way to relax mentally, and the allergic rashes had gone. Since then, I have discovered that my experience is by no means unusual. Other people with allergies have cured themselves in similar ways.

There was a bonus – I had found new friends. Many people who take up exercise in a regular way may continue all their lives, for all I know, as loners, daily ploughing up and down pools by themselves, running or cycling with only their own thoughts for company. Solitary exercise is in itself often attractive. It can be meditative and restful. But it's practically impossible to divorce yourself from your fellow exercisers all the time, even if you should wish to do so.

Exercise is one of the great common denominators among people, a forum where everybody is equal. It is the greatest social ice-breaker I know. And thus, apart from losing weight, improving my temper, building fitness and saying goodbye to medicaments, I discovered the friendships that build up at the poolside.

Anybody who has been in a pool at an appropriate time of day will confirm that swimmers talk together when not swimming. And it was this obvious contact between people that broadened my interest in the less measurable benefits of exercise. Watching middle-aged men and women, and even elderly people, at swimming pools, I was struck by the youthful quality of nearly all of them. They seemed mentally alert, possessed a clear love of life and, on top of all this, had the time to stop and talk.

CHAPTER THREE

An Alarming Trend

The social benefits of swimming seemed to make exercise worthwhile. But what are the facts? What is the common ground? How can you know which is the best form of exercise?

The most influential book I have come across in seeking answers is *Aerobics* by an American doctor named Kenneth Cooper. Aerobics literally means 'with oxygen', and aerobic exercises are ones that create a demand in the body for oxygen without producing an intolerable oxygen debt. In this way, unlike sprinting for example, they can be continued for long periods. They produce, in short, a 'training' effect, and promote wonderful changes in the body.

Principally, aerobic exercises give you a more efficient heart and respiratory system. Cooper breaks down the effectiveness of other exercises quite simply: **1.** Those that tense muscles without producing movement or demanding appreciable amounts of oxygen. Known as isometric exercises, they have no significant effect on overall health. **2.** Those that tense muscles to produce movement, but without very much demand for oxygen. Known as isotonic exercises (weightlifting is an example), they have little training effect on the heart and lungs. **3.** Those that demand a lot of oxygen (like the sprinting already mentioned), but are over too quickly to produce a definite training effect. These are known as anaerobic exercises.

The best aerobic exercises are running, cycling and swimming done rhythmically. And the particular value of Cooper's book I found initially was that it enabled me to place a 'value' on my daily swimming. Many people say they are not so concerned that they desire to evaluate their exercise in this way. They regard it as a peculiarly American obsession. I am not so sure: *Aerobics,* first published in

1968, has sold some eight million copies in various editions, and been printed in 19 languages, including Russian. We must all *need* to know whether or not we are doing enough exercise, particularly if our aim is general overall fitness rather than competition. And Cooper's great contribution has been to provide a simple method of quantifying effort in exercise.

For example, after a while I was able to swim 1,000 yards in about 21 minutes. With Cooper's book and a points system he devised, I was able to 'measure' this. As a man in my forties, swimming that distance in that time, six days in every seven, I was totting up a weekly 63 points on his system. It was more than twice as many, according to Cooper, as I needed to maintain a good standard of fitness.

The points system was based initially by Cooper, a former track athlete, on the yardstick of running or walking a mile at various speeds and correlating them with oxygen consumption, since the amount of oxygen your body can process and consume during maximum physical work is a firm guide to fitness. Cooper's intensive laboratory experiments established that anyone who ran a mile six times a week in less than eight minutes was maintaining a good fitness category, because a mile that fast demanded an expenditure of 35 millilitres of oxygen per minute – which Cooper said 'produces a beautiful training effect if done daily, six times a week'. Using the 8-minute mile as a basis, and awarding it five points, Cooper was able to evaluate other oxygen-consuming activities and draw up charts for the whole exercise spectrum. And he made this point about weekly programmes: 'Any variation in the daily routine is permissible as long as the week averages out to 30 points. Five days at six points per day is best. Four days at $7\frac{1}{2}$ points is a good happy medium. Three days at 10 points is still of value but you're close to the borderline (of fitness) because four days of nothing, out of seven, is a lot of nothing.'

Cooper nevertheless showed that quantity is not necessarily the determining factor. You can do less swimming than I do and still achieve a good standard of fitness. In fact, once you start exercising, you tend to find your own level of frequency. People who exercise more than most are almost certainly doing so because they enjoy it. If they are not, then they are misguided and are bound to give it up.

Clearly, what you want to know is the minimum level of exercise you need to do to keep fit. You tend to discover this for yourself because your body tells you. But in *New Aerobics*, published in 1970, Kenneth Cooper provides exercise scales according to age groupings, and in *Aerobics for Women*, written with his wife Mildred and published in 1972, he provides charts for women. The minimum basic target in each book nevertheless remains the same, about 30 points a week. This means for instance, that swimming 1,000 yards three times a week in a time below 25 minutes is just about as much as a man in his mid-forties needs to do to keep in good shape, providing the sessions are spaced reasonably evenly through the week.

The important point to remember is Cooper's insistent emphasis on the maintenance of heart and lung fitness. He best illustrates the importance of this in an anecdote in his first book. It is the true story of three men who volunteered for a special military project requiring the best possible physical condition. Of the three, one did not exercise regularly, one cycled about six miles a day going to and from his base and one did isometrics and weightlifting for an hour five days a week. The latter possessed a definitely muscular build, while the other two had normal builds. On an exercise treadmill, however, the muscular man, as well as the non-exerciser, were fatigued within five minutes, while the cyclist was still going strong 10 minutes later. He was the one recommended for the project.

That story shows what fitness really is. To many people, it simply means strength. But it is much more than this: it includes 'endurance', as Cooper's cyclist demonstrated.

Proper physical fitness, indeed, allows you to work without undue fatigue. It also leaves you with enough energy to tackle your hobbies and other recreational activities and to make maximum use of your body. And fitness includes your ability to fight infection, your freedom from disease

25

and being capable of meeting unexpected emergencies.

Fitness comes from regularly exercising all the muscles, the heart and the lungs, plus the skeleton and nervous system, which in turn improves the blood circulation and carries necessary nourishment to body cells. And it means becoming more aware of your own body's signals. Many unfit people get into trouble when they unexpectedly have to extend themselves physically, because they have dulled, if not actually erased, the warning signals which go to the fit person's brain.

This problem, one that applies to many people – all those, for example, who spend too much time watching television – was pinpointed by Bruce Tulloh, who ran for Britain and, after retiring in 1967, two years later set a record for running from Los Angeles to New York City: 'The majority of people over 30, and many of those over 20, have so far lost the fitness of childhood that they cannot even remember what it was like.'

Tulloh went on to tell people what fitness *does* feel like in a book he wrote on the subject: 'It is the feeling of lightness, of spring in your step when you walk down the road. It is the feeling of wondering what is round the next corner and not being afraid of it. It is being able to work all day, come home and go for a five-mile, half-hour run and feel refreshed by it; then to spend an hour in the garden, go to a dinner party, have a bottle of wine, dance, make love and wake up next morning looking forward to the day.'

The pity is that this still seems to be so little understood and appreciated. Meanwhile, disease of the coronary arteries and heart continues as the biggest killer in the Western world, accounting for something like twice the number of deaths as cancer. Even worse, coronary heart disease, lung cancer and cirrhosis of the liver are increasingly destroying people in the very prime of their lives. Of these, coronary heart disease poses the worst problem. In Britain, nearly 50 per cent of men who die before they reach the age of 65 do so because of diseases of the heart and circulation.

One of the problems in trying to reverse this alarming

26

trend, it often seems, is the attitude of some sections of the medical profession and their current predisposition, under the onslaught of advertising, to prescribe drugs. In fact, Britain's National Health Service drugs bill has doubled since 1967, costing the country £596 million in 1977, with about £4 million spent on slimming pills alone! A campaign is now in being to try to slice something off the total figure, powered by posters proclaiming: 'Be prepared to leave this surgery empty-handed.'

Certainly, fashions come and go in medicine, but before the advent of so many aids, and so many drugs, the old-fashioned family doctor was not above telling his patients simply to get some fresh air and exercise. He would tell you it was unlikely to do any harm, and it was always more likely to do a power of good. Doctors who are still convinced of the value of exercise rarely say much more than that it can help make your life more enjoyable. They don't say it will extend your life, only that it will add life to the years.

As to coronary heart disease, the basic arguments and divisions are best illustrated by those that surrounded a well-known study of London Transport workers which showed that bus drivers had more heart attacks than conductors did. Some experts suggested that the immunity of conductors was related to the running up and down stairs they do. Others that people prone to heart attacks, over-weight men for example, were those actually attracted to driving.

But there is sufficient statistical evidence now to make a compelling enough case in favour of taking aerobic exercise. One review of studies which relate physical activity and coronary heart disease, listed 13 retrospective analyses. They ranged from the one among London Transport men to another which studied San Francisco longshoremen (dockers). The total number of men covered came to nearly 200,000, and the relationship between lack of physical activity and coronary heart disease was borne out in all but two studies, one of these encompassing a small number of former oarsmen and another a small number of athletes.

27

While the connection with coronary heart disease was not demonstrated in these latter two, what was interesting was the fact that the oarsmen and athletes lived longer than their non-active contemporaries.

Another study, of 17,000 former students of Harvard University, not included in the aforementioned 13 analyses, showed that there were far fewer heart attacks among those who engaged regularly in activities like jogging, swimming, tennis and mountain climbing, than among those who were less active. In this study, questionnaires were sent in 1962 and 1966 to more than 36,000 men who had entered Harvard between 1916 and 1950. Questionnaires were sent out again in 1972 to the 16,936 men who returned the earlier questionnaires and declared themselves to be free of any known heart disease. It was discovered that in the interval there had been 572 heart attacks among them, 357 non-fatal and 215 fatal. The former students were asked about their daily amount of stair-climbing, walking, light sports activity and strenuous sports activity. This information was compiled into an index of physical activity expressed in calories expended each week. Those on the low side of this index, expending fewer than 2,000 calories a week, had a 64 per cent higher risk of a heart attack than their more energetic classmates. And it was calculated that if all the men had been on the high side of the index, 166 fewer heart attacks (86 non-fatal, 80 fatal) would have occurred in the study period.

From the Greeks to John F. Kennedy

Whether or not it is proved totally that heart disease can be substantially allayed by exercise, nobody seriously disputes that uncompetitive physical activity can provide useful relaxation of the type that anybody from a London bus driver to a busy executive or housewife might benefit from.

Unfortunately, what debate about the studies I mention did was to obscure the need to re-educate people about exercise. It is now an emergency situation. In Europe, deaths from coronary heart disease total over one million a year – more than the entire mortality during the Black

Death, which was spread over several years and killed over one-fifth of the population of Europe. And in Britain alone, by 1975 half a million people a year were found to be suffering from coronary heart disease.

In 1975 the *Sunday Times* carried an article on a group of men and women who were clearly outside the mainstream of the population in that they considered regular exercise important for themselves. Tests at London's Cavendish Medical Centre confirmed how healthy and fit they were compared with most people, of whom the newspaper said: 'Smoking, overweight, taking no regular strenuous exercise at all, they move like lemmings to early, quite unnecessary physical deterioration or even death.'

Ironically, in a world where communications have improved to a point where we can watch events in other countries as easily as the people who live there, an important message had not got across the Atlantic from the USA. There, since 1960, deaths from heart disease have dropped as a result of an increased awareness of the problem. Many Americans have been concerned enough to take up exercise, give up smoking (or smoke cigarettes that have less lethal contents) and to change their eating habits. In a similar period, deaths from heart disease in Britain have increased by a staggering 40 per cent.

How did this disparity occur? In truth, America was shaken years back. Studies comparing the fitness of America's youngsters with those of other countries, demonstrated how physically flabby they were. Even more, President Dwight D. Eisenhower's own cardiologist, the late Paul Dudley White, drew attention to the low standard of physical fitness among American adults. 'The greatest challenge of public and private health today, and the most neglected,' said White, 'is that of physical fitness in middle-age. It transcends, I believe, the problem of health of both youth and senility. The laudable goal of improving the physical (and mental) health of our youth should have no age limit at any decade, but it ought to continue on where it is needed most all through life.'

Later, President John F. Kennedy expressed equal concern and established an organisation, now called the President's Council on Physical Fitness and Sports, to try to improve the national levels of physical fitness. He personally directed the US officers of the General Staff in the Pentagon to get out from behind their desks and exercise daily – or accept demotion. And though someone observed that none of the generals lost their stars, they all lost their paunches.

'Physical fitness is not only one of the most important keys to a healthy body,' wrote Kennedy at the time, 'it is the basis of dynamic and creative intellectual activity. The relationship between the soundness of the body and the activities of the mind is subtle and complex. Much is not yet understood. But we do know what the Greeks knew – that intelligence and skill can function at the peak of their capacity only when the body is healthy and strong; that hardy spirits and tough minds usually inhabit sound bodies.

'The strength of our democracy is no greater than the collective well-being of our people. The vigour of our country is no stronger than the vitality and well-being of all our countrymen.'

Thus the national consciousness of the need for physical fitness was awakened in the USA at the very highest level.

CHAPTER FOUR

Time for Action

While the United States was waking up to the problems created by lack of physical exercise, the British remained complacent. To some extent, the complacency at one time was justified. We were still benefiting from wartime rationing, which had given us all a nutritionally well-balanced diet. Our schools still insisted on a stricter regimen of physical education. What's more, our schoolchildren were more often expected then to walk or cycle to and from school. Young men went into National Service, and if the schools failed to produce a good standard of physical fitness, the chances were that the Navy, Army or Air Force would redress the balance. We also introduced a National Health Service that was the envy of the world.

Then these beneficial factors started to be eroded away. The Health Service, intended to take care of us from womb to tomb, began to buckle under the demands made on it. An exploding drug industry helped divert doctors' attention from what was happening, until in the end some became merely prescription fillers. There was neither the time nor the energy to consider preventive medicine, which could have saved not only money but which would be, at its simplest, a matter of persuading people to walk round the block once a day.

In an effort to change the state of affairs, Britain's Health Education Council is now encouraging people to exercise, but repairing the omissions of more than a quarter of a century is a massive task. The battle against the pull of TV and the pub has barely begun.

One place where an impact has been made is Bath, which just happens to have a long history as a health centre. There, the district community physician, Dr. John Meadows, introduced fitness courses for men between 30 and 60 in the city's sports centre. The age-grouping encompasses men most at risk from coronary heart disease. They attend films and talks covering smoking, diet and the heart, and take part in supervised exercise sessions. Much of the exercise is done in the form of games similar to those played in gyms at school, and the middle-aged men who pay a small fee for the course appear to enjoy the games most of all. Some fun is thus immediately put back into their lives with physical fitness.

The long-term effects have yet to be seen, but the short-term ones are encouraging. Course members have cut down on smoking, or given it up altogether, have amended their diets and lost weight, and above all have started exercising. Many of them have taken to swimming regularly in the sports centre's pool.

Several men who have taken part in courses at Bath have done so following a coronary thrombosis. They have attended with the encouragement and *permission* of their family doctors. This altered attitude on the part of sections of the medical community is recent. And not all doctors even now approve of exercise as early as others.

Another place where exercise *is* employed in treatment is the King's Mill hospital at Sutton-in-Ashfield, Nottinghamshire, where the consultant physician is Dr. Roger Lloyd-Mostyn, who is one of a group of swimmers I report on later in this book. Dr. Lloyd-Mostyn encourages his patients to walk one or two miles a day only a week after a heart attack. A month later he checks their heart performance with a resting ECG (electrocardiogram) and, provided there are no disturbing results, an exercise ECG. If this also shows a satisfactory reading, then his patients attend once a week for six weeks for training in a gym. There they do 'circuit' training which includes sit-ups, skipping and working with medicine balls. At the end of the course they have a final check ECG.

The most telling effect of the exercise is psychological: it convinces the patients they are not 'dead'. As at Bath, the King's Mill patients are also given talks. Primarily, what the hospital hopes is that its patients will not only continue to exercise, but change to a wholly more healthy lifestyle than they had before.

People's own love of life is crucial in persuading them of the value of fitness. Without that there can be no hope of an interest in fitness being sustained or becoming self-generating. For example, it was a reader of the *Sunday Times* who, after seeing our feature story in 1975 on the middle-aged people who were fit, wrote with an idea. Why didn't the newspaper collect a group of more typical and generally 'unfit' middle-aged 'guinea pigs', he asked, and put them on a schedule of exercise, testing them before and after.

The *Sunday Times* decided to take up the idea, and the series that followed turned into a campaign with the slogan: Middle-age Fitness – Time for Action. Admired by both the Sports Council and the Health Education Council, it was like the old Charles Atlas ads but, instead of turning seven-stone weaklings into he-men, the newspaper went to work on the muscle that is the heart.

The *Sunday Times*'s experiment was neither large enough nor carried out on a sufficiently qualitative basis to have the broad validity scientists would accept. But, over two years, factors both encouraging and disturbing emerged from the study of the 12 men and women we selected.

When first tested, for instance, four of the 12 were found – when examined by exercise ECG taken while walking on a treadmill platform – to have some form of heart 'condition' which could have manifested itself clinically later in life, or more immediately if strenuous exercise was taken indiscriminately. 'Obviously,' the newspaper wrote at the time, 'this has serious implications for all of the middle-aged population, indicating a powerful argument for *prevention before cure.*'

As a result of the discovery, the four guinea pigs affected were streamed separately. They were called the Proceed-With-Caution group. The other eight formed the newspaper's Flat-Out group, and of these, four chose swimming as part of their exercise programme.

Two of the Proceed-With-Caution group also chose

swimming, and four months after the experiment's start the four 'worrying' cases were re-tested as an interim measure to see if they could go on to a more demanding exercise schedule. The test showed that all four had positively improved. One of them, an airline pilot whose first exercise ECG had shown a 'minor pattern change', was now entirely normal. 'It really is incredible,' he said. He had been running and cycling, and taking a collapsible bike with him on trips overseas.

Another of the Proceed-With-Caution group, a social scientist, had been shown to have a heart 'condition' which would always require caution, but swimming had begun to provide him with satisfying enjoyment in the mornings. It had also begun to help him handle the rest of the day better. 'I'm at a period in life (early fifties) which does tend to cause depression,' he said, 'and I have recently been feeling less depressed and more cheerful.'

The best thing that ever happened

Surprisingly, after almost a year, only one of the guinea pigs had dropped out of the programme. And when the *Sunday Times* re-tested the remaining 11, it was a success story. Individually, everybody's figures showed their heart to be operating more efficiently and comfortably, with a dramatically improved recovery after physical effort. There was also a significant reduction in the undesirable bloodstream fat called cholesterol, which in excess amounts is associated with increased incidence of coronary thrombosis.

The cholesterol reduction was particularly interesting, because up to that point, it had not been generally accepted – and may still not be – that exercise in itself will lower cholesterol levels. What *is* widely accepted by the medical profession is that a low-fat diet will lower cholesterol level by up to 20 per cent. However, all but one of the guinea pigs said they had remained on their normal diet after starting the programme, though they may have 'tended to eat less without deciding to' in some cases.

34

The difference in heart performance was explained thus by *Sunday Times* writer Norman Harris: 'Imagine that you are climbing five flights of stairs; or hurrying towards a bus stop; or digging the garden. And your heart is pumping furiously, your pulse is racing at about 160. You might even be provoking a heart attack. Now imagine that you have a twin beside you engaging in exactly the same activity, but instead of being 160, your twin's pulse is only 140. And that difference between the two of you has been brought about simply by a period of regular exercise. This is, in effect, what happened to our guinea pigs.'

Approximately a year on, the guinea pigs were tested once more. The *Sunday Times* had not been in touch with them since the end of the experiment, and so they were caught unawares. The results focused attention, as we wanted, on the long-term problem for anyone exercising – the question of motivation. Where our guinea pigs had kept up their exercising, swimming, jogging, cycling or even climbing up and down stairs, performance in the same tests were as good, if not better, than before. An example was a Welsh grocer who, two years before, had been pronounced 'basically unfit'. He was still running, was swimming and had also bought an indoor-exercise bike. 'The programme was the best thing that ever happened to me,' he said. 'I certainly didn't think so to start with, but I now realise it's essential; it's definitely become part of my life.' On his forest run, he was by now doing 24 minutes on a course which once took him 36 minutes.

Among those guinea pigs who had not kept up exercising to the same level, there was a measurable fall-back. One, for example, who had previously been a member of the Flat-Out group, had an exercise ECG result similar to that which the airline pilot had originally recorded and then rectified.

The pilot, having been shocked into action, had not given up at all. Indeed, when he first became a *Sunday Times* guinea pig, his airline medical rating had required him to have an ECG taken every six months. By now it was a statutory once-a-year test, the more frequent requirement having been rescinded as a result of his clear improvement in cardiac fitness.

On the whole, in fact, the guinea pigs had held their own. But only just. The question the re-testing posed was: Will people keep exercising when they do not face the possibility of a very public examination? It is still unresolved.

CHAPTER FIVE

This Fellow Feeling

Swimming pools are places where people are thrown together in a relaxed atmosphere. There is nothing like taking most of their clothes off to encourage people to behave naturally! Inhibitions are forgotten, and pomposities are cast away. It is very difficult to be anything but yourself when stripped down to swimwear. As a result, informal groups of acquaintances frequently operate within swimming pools.

A good example of how such a group works is provided by Gerald Forsberg, of whom there is more in this book, and who once swam the English Channel in a record time. He is now 65 and told me: 'Every day I go to Lancaster swimming bath. I swim with two people. I only know them there. I don't know them outside. I find their company enjoyable. We swim together for 50 lengths or so. You have the feeling of companionship. We never speak. There is a slight edge of competition; you don't want to be dragging along behind. There is this tremendous ensuing pleasure, this fellow feeling that you are doing something quite different to your ordinary work, and you're getting a tremendous mental relaxation because your work has absolutely disappeared from your mind. I've found I lead a completely different life for one hour a day. I haven't a clue what my companions do in outside life, but we just like to meet each other at the pool. All your worries disappear.'

The warm intimacy of a swimming pool is something of which Forsberg has had considerable experience. Two days after his record Channel swim, he was swimming up and down in the pool of the Royal Automobile Club in London, when another member said to him: 'I see you do a lot of swimming, and enjoy it. Do you mind if I give you a couple

37

of tips?' Forsberg, being a modest man, nodded, and received the following advice: 'If you didn't roll so much and if you didn't bend your knees at the back, I think you'd do reasonably well.' When Forsberg related this anecdote at his swimming club annual dinner that year, the members cheered and said: 'Quite right.'

Swimming pools, you see, are not only places where groups of people gather together easily, but places where advice is likely to be given freely, and received with considerable good humour. They are, for these reasons alone, ideal places for anybody to start getting fit, even if he or she plans to do something else more regularly later on.

A swimming pool is a haven, offering *protection*, particularly for people who are embarrassed by their shape and lack of fitness. Stripped down and in swimwear, you are no longer odd. If you don't believe this, try sitting fully clothed among swimmers of all shapes and sizes on a poolside in the summer sun. *You* will be the one who feels strange.

In my experience, children and adults never make fun of fat or elderly people in pools. Fatness *sometimes* tends to be associated with swimmers. It may have something to do with newspaper pictures of long-distance swimmers who like a layer of fat to help them keep warm in cold water. And though most regular swimmers are reasonably slim, a bit of blubber in a swimming pool is more likely to command respect than attract ridicule.

If you *are* fat, the water will help to get you fit more comfortably than exercise on land, because it will support your weight. That support also means swimming is particularly beneficial to people with injuries and who suffer from back trouble, though they should stay away from the butterfly stroke, because it forces the body to arch backward. Weightlessness in the water also makes swimming an especially good activity for elderly people. And because the body is like a boat when it comes to moving through the water, older people can find solace in the fact that smooth strokes can counterbalance a great deal of any loss of strength.

As a therapeutic exercise, swimming is unequalled, bringing gently back into action muscles perhaps severely atrophied by lack of use; and it is an activity that can be practised by handicapped people. No sight is nearer and dearer to the hearts of those who defend the cost of swimming pools, than people who might otherwise not be able to exercise effectively, experiencing the unimpeded joy of moving through the water. Swimming improves anyone's flexibility.

If you are interested in body-strength, swimming also exercises the shoulders more, perhaps, than any sport except weightlifting, and it strengthens the legs. For a woman, the fact that swimming tends to build long rather than short, knotted muscles, is a particular advantage. But perhaps swimming's greatest attraction is that, like no other physical activity, it offers an unlimited possibility of exercise without the danger inherent in body-contact sport, or the joint, bone and muscle problems that plague runners, tennis players and gymnasts.

In terms of improving heart and lung efficiency, and losing weight, it is difficult to compare swimming with other activities, but according to Kenneth Cooper it comes a close second to running. He says: 'The big advantage of swimming is that, for most people, it is much more enjoyable than running.' Simply going to the water to exercise is among the most natural things we can do.

The origins of man go back to the water, where all life began, and George Leonard, in a book called *The Ultimate Athlete*, discusses the significance of this: 'Through the mysterious process of evolution, we have somehow learned to enclose . . . the wild and varied life of the sea within our own bodies. We may walk upright on dry land but we can never escape the sea. We must continually reconstitute its liquids and salts inside ourselves to keep alive organs that move with the unhurried peristaltic rhythms of the creatures that abound in the eternal waters. Even if the body itself, organs and all, should be transformed, its transformation would be in the nature of a sea change, inexorable and profound.'

This passage helps explain why people are so attracted to the sea and water. As an island nation, the British spend a great deal of time travelling to the coast. When we get there, even if we do not swim, we sit contemplating the sea at great length. Are we studying the rhythms of our own bodies by watching the waves and tides?

I think that in some way we are. Rhythm *is* crucial to our lives. There is a daily one and a yearly one. Our lives, by the week, by the month and the season are inexorably bound up in these natural factors. Life, from birth to death, is governed by an encompassing rhythm. If we recognise this we can lead distinctly healthier lives.

Is it so surprising that we feel so natural in water? It is at the source of everything. After all, we spend the first nine months of life in the warm, watery sac of the womb, and we are composed of water with chemicals.

Once in the water – up to your neck in it – you become one of a group of equals, joined by water. Nobody is taller or smaller than anyone else; children are level with adults, mother with father. The water indiscriminately provides physical and mental relaxation, and thus sustenance. As warm water in the winter's indoor pool divides and deluges the body's surfaces, and sparkling water cools the summer heat, it provides man and woman with one of the most sensuous experiences they can ever know. This is a child's delight, a home from home, that can be enjoyed until one's dotage. A luxurious, comfortable gymnasium in which gravity is defied, and the imagination is the only boundary.

What happens to the heart in that watery world of swimming is quite remarkable, and is explained next.

CHAPTER SIX

An Affair of the Heart

We all know the surprise we sometimes feel on discovering that somebody is either much younger or much older than we had guessed. In my childhood, it was quite common still to see working-class mothers who, bowed down with worry and undermined by a low standard of diet, often looked over 40 when they were still in their twenties. Though there are now fewer women like this, we are not without examples of premature physical ageing. Today, women and men can as easily age physically from too much food, too much tension and too little exercise.

Of the three, it is lack of physical exercise that is undoubtedly most responsible for premature ageing. This is because exercising helps to prevent tension and to burn up calories. In turn, experience shows that exercising leads to more sensible eating. As a result of being exercised, the body, moreover, does not wear out. We are not like cars; our bodies actually thrive on being used.

You might ask how we can be sure that this is so. The ultimate proof is provided by the unfortunate person who has to lie in bed for an extended period, say in a hospital ward. As he lies there, the muscles waste away, and the bones in time become brittle and thinner than normal. 'Lying rotting in bed' is a fact, not a fiction or a sergeant-major's fantasy designed to frighten slothful recruits.

Contrast this image with anybody you have ever known who exercises regularly. According to one doctor: 'Physical activity, and straining and tugging on bones, helps develop them no matter what the person's age. When you flex your muscles your bones become harder.' Older people who take up exercise can actually add weight and strength to their bones while building up and maintaining muscle. It is just as if exercise is an elixir of youth.

And if such processes of physiological maintenance provided by regular exercise can apply to muscle and bones, imagine what they mean for the heart! About the size of a fist, the heart is a muscular organ that starts beating regularly by the time we are four weeks old in the womb. We then depend on it never to cease working for us until the day we die. Yet the disregard some people have for it makes it little wonder that the heart in modern man and woman has begun more frequently to give up a battle of often unequal odds.

The odds are stacked against the heart by fatty deposits laid down in the lining of the major arteries. It is like rust collecting in a pipe. When the rust grows to a point where the passage of blood to the heart or brain is blocked, a heart attack occurs in the first case and a stroke in the second.

It is the penalty of living in a developed country: we age before our time if we fail to take precautions. The fact that the ageing process is not necessarily a chronological matter was dramatically observed in young Americans killed in the Korean War. There, autopsies demonstrated that fatty deposits were present in the arterial walls of 77 per cent of the dead men. Their average age was 22. Since most men do not achieve their physical maturity until 26, it meant that the young soldiers, as a result of diet and inadequate exercise, had bodies that had been deteriorating while still developing!

Scientists once believed that the laying down of fatty deposits in the arteries was not only inevitable, but irreversible. Recent evidence, however, suggests that the development of deposits in the arteries, at least in the early stages, can not only be halted, but even reversed, by exercise of the heart and lungs. 'There is probably a point beyond which the process does not reverse,' says one expert, 'but the important thing is that man may be more in control of his destiny than he thinks.'

But why is exercise so good for the heart? And for the lungs, which provide the fuel? The easiest way for the non-expert to understand is simply to compare the heart to a car engine. A more powerful car engine tackles a hill climb, for instance, with less effort than a smaller engine. It does something comfortably which a smaller engine can cope with only by operating at such a rate that it may be 'screaming' with effort. That may be all right as far as a small engine is concerned, but in the case of your own heart, which would you prefer? One that tackles tasks with reasonable ease, or one that 'screams' with effort?

A healthy heart in a human body with lungs used to some strenuous exercise is, like the large car engine, more powerful and efficient – and a heart can increase with exercise up to 15 per cent in size. It beats more slowly at rest and at work, acquires a greater pumping capacity and recovers more rapidly and smoothly from effort.

Thus, with a 'big-engine' heart, you are much more capable of meeting physical demands. In an emergency, or simply in one of those silly situations where you are suddenly involved in an unexpected physical game, it is far less likely to fail you.

Exercise not only strengthens the heart, it provides it with a support system, because every muscle is, in effect, a miniature heart, helping to pump blood. When a muscle contracts, it squeezes blood towards the heart; when it relaxes, it allows the muscle to be filled with blood, like the heart.

In other words, by exercising, you build up a whole army of hearts. This dramatically contrasts with the fat person, who not only has a smaller army but taxes the heart and its support system in an unfair way because fat contains millions of capillaries that need to be serviced with blood.

Authors Stephen Lock and Tony Smith list in the *Medical Risks of Life* some of the amazing things that happen when one exercises. The blood-flow, for example, may be 30 times faster than when one is at rest, the amount of oxygen used 100 times the resting value and the rise in temperature as much as two or three degrees centigrade. Blood is also switched from relatively inessential parts of the body, such as the intestines, to the general circulation. The flow to the skin may be increased by as much as four times, since both sweating and the generalised widening of the small blood vessels in the skin help to get rid of heat generated by exercise. And though the heart-rate speeds up less in the person who regularly exercises than in the person who does not, the amount of blood pumped out by the heart may be half as much again – 30–36 litres a minute, compared with 24 litres.

So effort is easier if you are fit. Anyone who has watched veteran runners sprinting for the tape, must suspect that this is the case. I say runners, rather than swimmers, simply because it is easier to see their faces, and therefore, to know whether or not they are competing capably. Naturally, what nags at the mind is the thought that somebody might die as a result of exertion when older. Death during exercise is, however, almost always due to a previously undiagnosed complaint.

When we first planned the series on middle-aged fitness in the *Sunday Times*, we contacted Dr. Sir Roger Bannister to express our concern for the risks of encouraging perhaps thousands of middle-aged and older people to go out and exercise. We had nightmare visions of men and women, prompted by us, going out to engage in strenuous physical activity perhaps for the first time in years, and promptly dropping dead. And further nightmares about the possible repercussions for the newspaper. Roger Bannister put our minds at rest. The risk, he said, was greater for these people if they did not exercise than if they did. Thus any risk we took, which was minimal, had to be worthwhile.

In all of this, the heart of the swimmer has a particular advantage which was first drawn to my attention by Dr. Ernst Jokl, an American specialist in physiology. Jokl compared the running and swimming world records after the Montreal Olympics in 1976, and showed that the decline of speed with distance is greater in running than in swimming, and that runners lose speed at rates almost three times greater than swimmers. Why should there be such a discrepancy?

Jokl said it was explained by recent research into weightlessness, a problem of major importance for space medicine. He cited, in particular, some remarkable X-ray pictures, obtained by Professor Otto Gauer of the University of Berlin. These showed the heart of a person upright, next supine and then horizontally buoyed up in water, and demonstrated that the cardiac volume increased from 689 millilitres to 771 millilitres when horizontal, and to 922 millilitres following immersion in water. With Professor Gauer's permission the drawings on pages 46–47 are based exactly on his photographs. They show more clearly, for the non-expert, how the heart size increases.

It *was* realised that the cardiac volume expands when the body is horizontal because of the more even distribution of blood through the body. But little awareness has existed of what occurs when the body is immersed in water. Nobody had thought to take X-rays. Such enlargement of the heart of a person immersed in water, however, means that 10 to 20 per cent more blood is expelled with each contraction compared with when one is running in a vertical position, supporting oneself against gravity. For the swimmer, the benefit is enormous, providing the potential to work harder, and for a longer period of time. It explains why long-distance swimmers can keep going for so long and so well, and why people with a lower-than-normal heart capacity can, in the water, exercise at a higher level than they can on land. It also provides an important part of the reason for the vastly improved performance of women in the water, where in long-distance swims these days they are often superior to men.

The water provides other advantages apart from a state of simulated weightlessness. There is the cooling effect of the water itself. This diverts blood from the skin to the central circulation, which in turn contributes to an increased capacity of the cardio-vascular system to carry oxygen to the muscles. And while the benefits provided by swimming to functional lung capacities have not been sub-

Overleaf: Illustrations based on X-ray photographs showing the change of heart size in relation to posture and immersion of a person in water. Drawings by Sidney Woods with the kind permission of Dr. Otto Gauer of the University of Berlin.

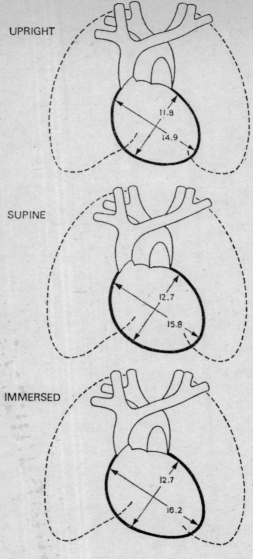

UPRIGHT

11.8
14.9

SUPINE

12.7
15.8

IMMERSED

12.7
16.2

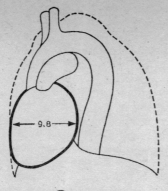

689 ml

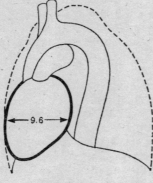

771 ml

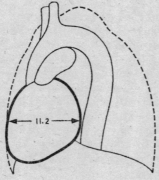

922 ml

47

stantiated by published research, Professor Paul Hutinger, writing in his own American publication called Master Swimmers Lane 4, compares swimmers with gymnasts at Western Illinois University to show that the swimmers have a higher lung capacity. Anything up to a fifth more. Hutinger has also reported a comparison of the lung capacity of veteran swimmers, from data taken at Western Illinois swim clinics, and a sample of veteran runners. Again the swimmers had a higher capacity.

Importantly, Hutinger compared the breathing pattern and technique used by swimmers with exercises given lung patients by therapists. These exercises usually include exhaling, or forcefully blowing out through pursed lips, which causes the lungs to push out air against a resistance, and helps to increase the functional ability of the lungs. Hutinger, a veteran champion himself, wrote that in swimming 'blowing out air against the resistance of the water is similar to therapy exercises. The controlled breathing and explosive exhalation during the 30-minutes to hour-long training sessions contributes to the high lung volumes observed in most veteran swimmers.'

Study of veteran swimming performances in America demonstrates the resulting effect. Men near 60 years of age can swim 70 per cent as fast as men in their twenties. Several men near 60 are breaking 60 seconds for the 100 yards freestyle. And overall, veterans who keep training show only a one per cent per year fall-off in performance over the period of middle-age. Perhaps part of the reason for the phenomenal increase in competitive swimming for 'veterans' from the age of 25 on (or Masters Swimming) has, as in veteran athletics from 40 on for men (35 for women), been due to the fact that those who take up training seriously for the first time in their lives during middle-age, often discover they can perform better than they did in their youth. It is this fascination, apart from the pursuit of good health, that is the only possible explanation for the growing popularity. In the USA today they have an estimated one million regular veteran swimmers, ranging in age from 25 to 80 years of age.

A Testing Time

Photographic report
by Chris Smith
of the testing of a
group of
veteran swimmers in
the human
performance laboratory
at St. Mary's College,
Twickenham

A full account of the tests and
results is given in Chapter Seven
starting on page 50

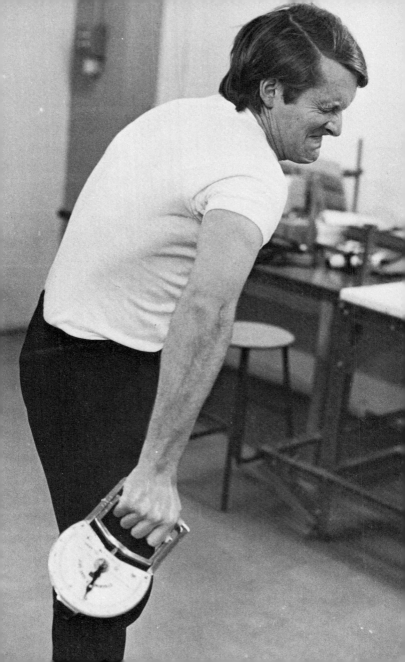

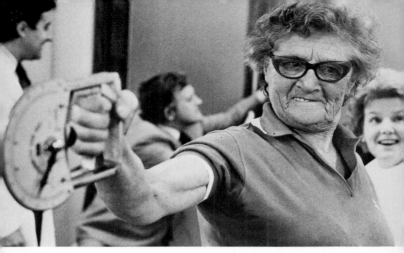

Charles Doxat, 35 (*opposite*), and Vivienne Cherriman, 70 (*above*), checked their grip strength in a test that is a good guide to general overall muscular strength. Cherriman gripped 55 lb with her right hand, Doxat 101 lb with his.

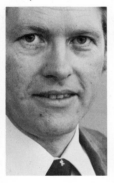

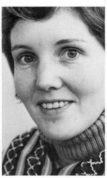

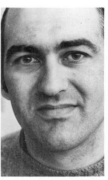

Bob Burn, 40 proved fitter than average man of his age, earned the commendation: 'Still with it'. Demonstrated an impressive respiratory efficiency.

Barbara Williamson, 39, after having three children and now working in a sedentary job, showed she remains 'a good physical specimen'.

James Stewart, 35, had polio, suffered from asthma when younger, and now committed to a demanding career, uses swimming to keep fit.

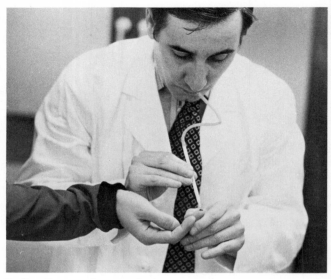

Dudley Cooper, who supervised tests, obtained blood samples using pipette (*above*) and measured the haemoglobin content (*below*) using a photometer.

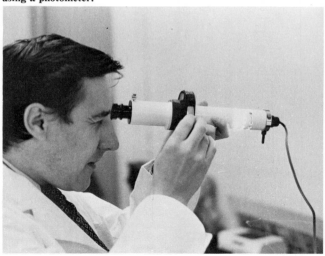

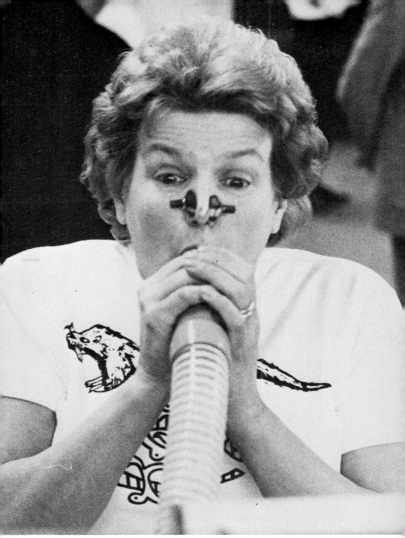

Lillian Bell, 47, blew into a dry spirometer to check her lung capacity and Forced Expiratory Volume, or the percentage of air that can be expelled in one second. Bell's capacity measured 3.55 litres and her FEV was 66 per cent, not bad for a former heavy smoker who now swims up to three hours a day.

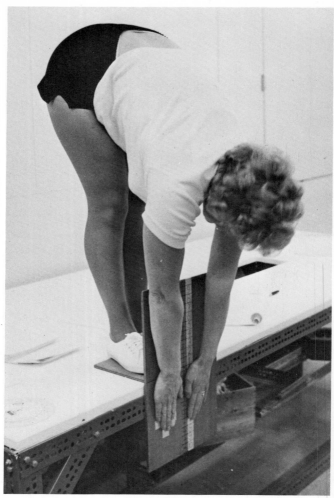

In the picture above, Lillian Bell demonstrates one of the three most remarkable flexibility performances among the women swimmers, reaching 16.5 cm below her toes. *Opposite:* Gerald Forsberg, 65, muses on the demands of the bicycle ergometer. He could not touch his toes but he did once swim the English Channel in a record time and he still swims vigorously practically every day.

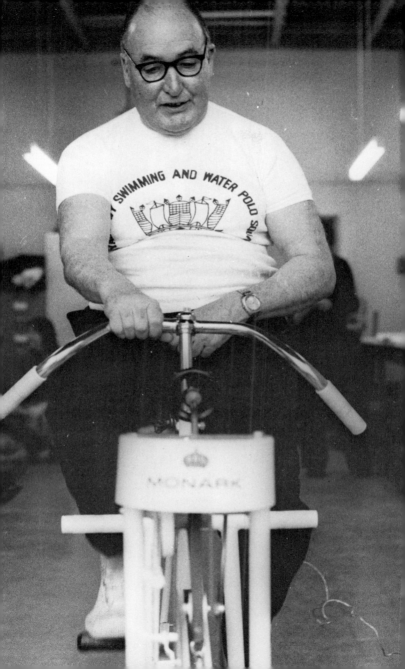

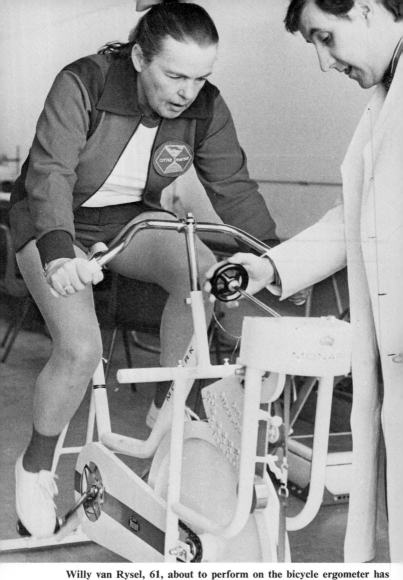

Willy van Rysel, 61, about to perform on the bicycle ergometer has the workload adjusted by Dudley Cooper. His verdict: 'She's an advertisement for exercise.'

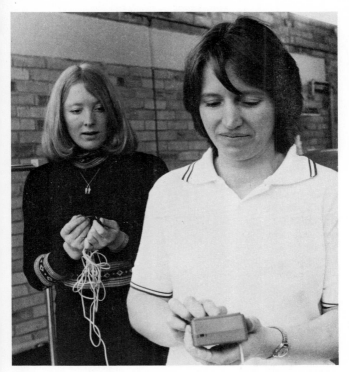

Lesley Nice, 32, averaged 0.227 sec in the reaction time test, which involved pushing a button as fast as possible each time a light came on. Most of the veteran swimmers retained reactions of 20-year-olds.

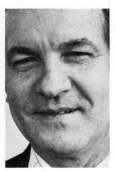

Ron Roberts, 56, (*left*), swam in two Olympics and claims, 'Swimming is a lot better than any medicine I ever had.'

Douglas Payne, 47, (*right*), a busy bank manager who still swims, 'scored better than expected.'

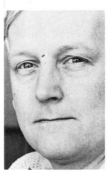

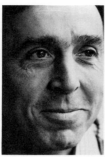

John Lovesey, 45, author of this book, swims up to five times a week. He earned commendation: 'Fit for his age.'

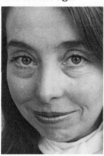

Vivenne Crowe, 40, who once swam for England, proved she is ticking over nicely for a woman who once gained a surplus of four stone in weight.

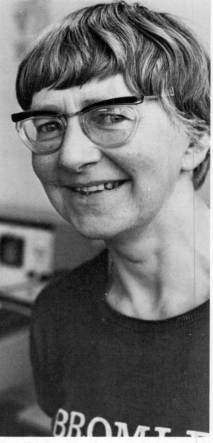

Betty Condon, 55, swims up to six days a week. A widow, she is, said St. Mary's College, a remarkable example of how physical recreational activity can help somebody overcome life's traumas.

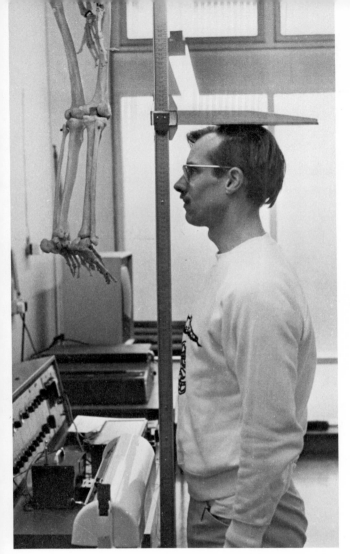

Dr. Roger Lloyd-Mostyn, 36, is a consultant physician at a Nottinghamshire hospital where post-coronary cases are helped to recovery with exercises. He practises what he preaches: Lloyd-Mostyn proved to be one of the fittest veteran swimmers tested.

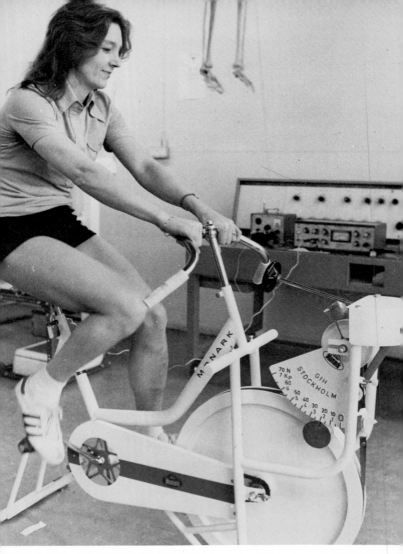

Jean Chipperfield, 37, improved her health by taking up swimming and first swam competitively at 36. She is proof, commented St. Mary's College, that it is never too late to start. It is a picture of her on the cover of this book.

In Britain, the way has been led by certain individual enthusiasts and by London's Otter Swimming Club, which has staged a Masters Tournament every year since 1972. The Amateur Swimming Association is planning the first national veterans' competition for 1979. Meanwhile, with the thought of providing positive proof of the value of regular swimming to the health and general enjoyment of life of people over 30, I arranged for some male and female swimmers from the Otter tournament to be tested in the Human Performance Laboratory at St. Mary's College, Twickenham, Middlesex.

CHAPTER SEVEN
A Testing Time

'Actually I felt somewhat ashamed of my weak effort in the "vital capacity" test. I really was surprised it was so poor. However, I feel pretty fit, and can't grumble at my age. Your comments were pleasant, and I thank you for your good wishes for my hoped-for swim across the Solent in the summer. I believe you said Betty Condon could train harder, and Willy van Rysel should be best suited to the sprints – any help for me regarding actual workload swimmingwise?'

That passage is taken from a letter received at St. Mary's College after the tests were run on the veteran swimmers from the Otter tournament. It could be a letter from a youngster with perhaps a long-term eye on swimming the English Channel. The giveaway is the words 'can't grumble at my age'. Vivienne Cherriman was 70 at the time, and the two other women she refers to, 55 and 61 respectively.

At St. Mary's, the group ranged in age, men and women, from Mrs. Cherriman, who is from the Isle of Wight, down to Mrs. Lesley Nice, 32, from Dover. In competitive performance, the range went from Mrs. Jean Chipperfield, 37, who first took part in a swimming tournament in 1977, to 65-year-old Commander Gerald Forsberg, whose time for swimming the Channel from England to France, 13 hours 33 minutes, was a record in 1957; and 57-year-old Ron Roberts, who swam for Britain in the 1952 and 1956 Olympics.

There were eight women and seven men from the Otter tournament, and to even up the numbers and discover what I was asking them all to submit to, I took the tests myself. The group included a civil servant, an advertising company executive, a bank clerk, a personnel officer, a consultant physician, a security executive and an author. With one exception, each held down a job at the time of the tests, and all their posts were demanding in terms of both time and responsibility. Even Mrs. Cherriman, at 70, was still working, as a senior lecturer in law, six hours a day, four days a week. And she has had six children.

Some of the younger women, apart from coping with a full-time job, were bringing up children and running a home, with no apparent strain. One of the older women was managing her own home and looking after her elderly parents in another, 'running two homes and two gardens', as she said. Their commitments ensured that the time spent in training by the swimmers in the group in any one week was unexceptional. Anyone who claimed they could not possibly emulate them, in terms of time spent, would have to be either grossly overworked or just plain lazy.

The fact that a majority in the group said they engaged in some form of physical activity daily did not mean they were hellbent on swimming seven days a week, 52 weeks a year. Far from that, time spent in the pool was sometimes of the order of once a week, though most managed a minimum of two or three times. The most striking common characteristic of the group was that they were not simply energetic, but generally involved in a whole host of activities in addition to swimming. These ranged from playing golf to felling trees.

Strikingly, with one exception, they all listed a second sporting interest, the women mentioning hockey, netball, badminton or table tennis, the men rugby, running, golf, football or cricket. Moreover, though all still competed in swimming, sometimes only once or twice a year, a majority emphasised that they swam primarily for both pleasure and physical health reasons. Only two of the women said they took part in swimming to gain competitive success.

It was an intriguing consensus – the general agreement that they swam largely for pleasure – considering that the group contained more than one swimmer who had competed for their country. But it bears out the point that competitive success in middle-age and even older is most important to people who have not had an opportunity to enter tournaments before.

Attitudes to ageing, in fact, have so drastically altered in the past 10 or 20 years that it is conceivable that women like Mrs. Cherriman will soon not be uncommon. Mrs. Cherriman was born, after all, in an era when physical sporting activity among females was likely to be frowned on in many families. One of the group, Willy van Rysel, was born in Holland into just such a family. Her mother disapproved of girls going swimming, so Willy, a resourceful youngster, used to swim wearing just a long vest made respectable with a safety-pin. Going home she would swing the vest in the air to dry it, and then put it on at the last moment in a ladies' convenience, before arriving home to her unsuspecting mother.

The diversity of interest and, to some extent, of social class, evident within the group, is typical of swimming. Like running and other individual activities, it appears to attract self-sufficient, socially mobile, aware people. 'It cannot be by chance,' said Dudley Cooper, head of the Movement Studies Department at St. Mary's College, 'that two highly individual sports, like swimming and running, cater for such a wide range of the population. Rugby caters for a relatively small social strata, affected only by the part of the country you are in. Soccer does also at another level, though it has attempted to break down class barriers. Tennis is still a very much middle-class game, and the problem accordingly posed is epitomised probably best of all in the golf club: the problem of getting in. People never have any problem getting into a swimming club. You don't have to have references. They're just delighted to have you.'

On the day of the tests at St. Mary's College, the most immediately observable common characteristic among the group was the ability of them all to get on with each other. A pool attendant (two of the women worked in this capacity) was able to talk to a man who had been a deputy director with the Ministry of Defence. A man of 36 was able to talk to a woman twice his age in a conversation that went considerably beyond polite chit-chat. What they had in common was swimming, and the social ease which is quite evidently associated with that activity. Afterwards

Mrs. Cherriman said: 'The tests were interesting, and apart from that the social climate was great, and it was enjoyable meeting up with other swimmers.' Crucially, each member of the group was obviously enjoying life.

The human performance laboratory at St. Mary's College can be used to measure everything, from the time it takes a woman or man to react to a visual signal to the performance of the heart under stress. Some of the footballers in England's national team have been there – the laboratory discovered that one of them could not even touch his toes – and so have athletes like David Bedford and New Zealand's Olympic champion, John Walker. Later the same day as the veteran swimmers were tested, members of Britain's national rowing squad had a similar performance rule run over them.

Human performance laboratories are not a new phenomenon, but it is true to say their use has been longer recognised in the USA, Scandinavia and Eastern Europe than in Britain. Their value lies in two areas. Firstly, in the long-term collection of information about sportspeople and (when they can be persuaded to be tested) less physically able people, with all the lessons that can be learned to the benefit of the population generally. And secondly, in the opportunity such laboratories provide competitors for assessment, and thereby guidance about everything from training to the activities for which they may be best suited.

At St. Mary's, Dudley Cooper, both a physical educationist and an exercise physiologist, who is in charge of the human performance laboratory, agreed it would be valuable to test a group of middle-aged people who swam regularly, particularly since very little research has been carried out on swimmers after an age at which they give up normal open competition. It is generally acknowledged that swimming helps to sustain and improve health, but measurement of the benefits have not often been attempted.

With this thought in mind, Dudley Cooper decided that each swimmer in the group would be subjected to the following examination:

1. A blood test to measure haemoglobin content. Haemoglobin is the protein in red blood cells which transports oxygen to the tissues. A good average haemoglobin content might measure anything from 13 to 17 grams per 100 millilitres. But as our tests showed, women often have a lower red blood cell content, and thus tend to be handicapped in sporting performances because they simply cannot carry as much oxygen as men. Many pre-menopausal women, in particular, are chronically iron deficient because they do not easily replace the monthly blood loss. Moreover such mild anaemia is not easily noticed, and that is why Joan Ullyot, a medical doctor and competitive athlete in America who has become well-known for her writing on the subject of women and exercise, says: 'I think all women should take a daily iron supplement to make sure their bodies will manufacture as many red cells as possible.'

2. A grip-strength test of both hands, used separately. A good indication this, of general overall muscular strength, taking into account the general body-build of the subject.

3. A simple reaction-time check, the implications of which are anything *but* simple, in which the subject pushes a button as soon as possible after a light comes on. A gauge of visual aptitude and reflex ability, the results demonstrated that people who regularly exercise suffer surprisingly little loss in this area. Most 20-year-olds would have a reaction time between 0·200 sec and 0·250 sec. The swimmers' awareness and rapid reactions account in part for their continuing enjoyment of life. As somebody once pointed out to me, we do not just feed ourselves through our mouths, but with all our senses. Food for the mind is provided partly by food for the eyes.

4. A measurement taken of the vital capacity, or the amount of air that can be exhaled after a full inhalation. The functional lung capacity of a 50-year-old is usually 35 per cent less than that of a person of 30. However, regular swimmers in particular tend to reverse or slow down such deterioration. You can judge how well from the vital capacities of those tested, whose results should be compared with say, the average capacity of a man of 49, which is likely to be no more than three litres.

5. And still with the lungs, a measurement of the FEV, which stands for Forced Expiratory Volume, or the percentage of air contained in the lungs that can be expelled in one second. The familiar comment: 'You've got a good pair of bellows!' to someone who has just blown out the candles on a birthday cake, explains what this test is all about. You cannot expel 98 per cent of the air in your lungs in one second, as one of our swimmers did, without being very fit in terms of the muscles that control the operation.

6. An exercise ECG (electrocardiogram) to test the functional ability of the heart while pedalling a bicycle ergometer on which the workload can be increased according to the subject. The heart of a person who regularly exercises can attain a greater work capacity with a lower heart rate than that of someone who does not take part in physical activity. However, to understand the figures for the exercise heart rates at maximum effort that were obtained at St. Mary's, one needs to know the gradual decline of maximum heart rate with age. Many young swimmers, for example, reach heart rates of 220 per minute and the approximate decline is as follows: 20–30 years old – a maximum heart rate of 200; 31–40 – maximum 190; 41–50 – maximum 180; 51–60 – maximum 170.

Derived from the performance on the bicycle is another figure given in the results – VO2. This is a measure of oxygen uptake in millilitres per kilogram of the individual weight, over the period of a minute. It is simply an indication of the ability of the body to deliver oxygen to its various parts. Average male college students measured in America produced figures from 41 to 48 ml/kg/min. But in studying the figures for the swimmers tested at St. Mary's, one needs to account for the fact that swimmers tested on an ergometer will usually have a lower oxygen uptake than they would if tested in the water, because of the difference in the exercise. It amounts to a difference of about 5 ml/kg/min.

7. A measurement of flexibility or the maintenance of mobility in the joints, as a result of exercise – a 'toe-touching' test in which the object is to measure how far beyond the toes the subject, standing above floor level, can stretch. You will see that the women were generally much more flexible than the men.

8. A check on height and weight, from which was obtained the Rating of Ponderal Index (RPI), a measure merely of fatness. The higher the figure, the leaner the subject.

In addition to the tests, our subjects filled in questionnaires covering everything from sporting history to their record of illness and job responsibility. For all of them it was a low point in the year, winter, and they were doing less swimming perhaps than in the summer. However, one would be hard put to find people, of similar ages, as fit as they were among the general run of the population at any time. The results:

WOMEN

Lesley Nice. From Dover, Kent, aged 32, married, two children, working as a pool attendant, helps to run Dover Lifeguard Club. Competed for Middlesex Schools swimming team, took up swimming again to lose weight, now swims about three times a week. Second best sport: hockey, but no longer plays.

St. Mary's College comment: Not fat, reasonably strong, reasonably flexible with a reasonable reaction time. Her respiratory function is not bad and, at 32, she is capable of improvement. A clear case of a woman who, having kept her fitness topped up while coping with two young children, is now capable of managing a more vigorous exercise programme if she wishes.

TEST RESULTS. Height: 5 ft 7 in. Weight 9 st 13 lb. RPI: 12·80. Grip strength: Right hand – 89 lb. Left hand – 96 lb. Flexibility: 5·1 cm. Simple reaction time – 0·227 sec. Haemoglobin (g/100 ml): 11·0. Vital capacity (litres): 3·80.

FEV: 94%. Exercise heart rate (bpm): 160. VO2 (ml/kg/min): 32·00. Smokes: No. Drinks alcohol: occasionally.

Jean Chipperfield. From Shoreham-by-Sea, Sussex, aged 37, married, three children, working as a pool attendant and swimming instructor. First swam competitively at 36, and achieved her best performance at 37. Now swims almost daily.

St. Mary's College comment: Though not particularly strong, she is a pretty fit person for her age group, and could take part in most activities without strain. She has good flexibility, reaction time and lung capacity. What is interesting about her, is that she is living proof that it is never too late to start. She has only taken up swimming, more seriously, in the past two years, and is still improving.

TEST RESULTS. Height 5 ft 4 in. Weight: 8 st 6 lb. RPI: 13·10. Grip strength: Right hand – 66 lb. Left hand – 66 lb. Flexibility: 15·2 cm. Simple reaction time 0·225 sec. Haemoglobin (g/100 ml): 13·8. Vital capacity (litres): 4·00. FEV: 88·5%. Exercise heart rate (bpm): 140. VO2 (ml/kg/min): 42·00. Smokes: 10 cigarettes a day. Drinks alcohol: occasionally.

Barbara Williamson. From Babbacome, Devon, aged 39, married, three children. Once a policewoman, she is now a bank clerk. A former national junior freestyle record-holder and a national lifesaving champion who represented Britain in an international lifesaving competition in 1971, she still swims three or four times a week. Second best sport: netball, but does not play very often nowadays because 'I've run out of time.'

St. Mary's College comment: A very strong girl who is big physically and was able to work at a higher load on the bicycle than the other women. What is a credit to her is that after having had three children and now working in a sedentary occupation, she has managed to maintain her fitness very well. At nearly 40, she is still a good physical specimen.

TEST RESULTS. Height: 5 ft 8½ in. Weight: 12 st 1 lb. RPI: 12·25. Grip strength: Right hand – 89 lb. Left hand – 77 lb. Flexibility: 16·5 cm. Simple reaction time 0·226 secs. Haemoglobin (g/100 ml): 11·5. Vital capacity (litres): 4·05. FEW 90%. Exercise heart rate (bpm): 135. VO2 (m/kg/min): 30·0. Smokes: No. Drinks alcohol: occasionally.

Vivienne Crowe. From Winchcombe, Gloucester, age 40, married, no children, working as a bank personnel officer. Swam backstroke for England in the 1954 Commonwealth Games in Vancouver. When she gave up competing at top level, she gained weight until she was four stones heavier than she is today. She trimmed down to her present figure by dieting, and keeps her weight constant by a mixture of physical activity and careful control of a normal diet. She exercises anything up to seven days a week, an hour on each occasion, but often by walking, not always by swimming. Second best sport: hockey, but has not played for a long time.

St. Mary's College comment: Her lung capacity is very good for her size. She has average strength, average flexibility and her reaction time is better than average. Her performance on the bicycle was quite good, and she is a generally competent, almost athletic, type who is ticking over and could, if she wished, probably perform even better.

TEST RESULTS. Height: 5 ft 5 in. Weight 9 st 4 lb. RPI: 12·80. Grip strength: Right hand – 74 lb. Left hand – 68 lb. Flexibility: 5·1 cm. Simple reaction time 0·194 sec. Haemoglobin (g/100 ml): 12·4. Vital capacity (litres): 3·65. FEV: 90·5%. Exercise heart rate (bpm): 145. VO2 (m/kg/min): 34·50. Smokes: No. Drinks alcohol: Occasionally.

Lillian Bell. From Knutsford, Cheshire, aged 47, married, three children, working as a sports centre attendant. A long-distance swimmer who competed for Preston, she stopped 18 years ago, but took to the water again two years ago. She now swims almost daily, usually for an hour but sometimes up to three hours to make up for any day missed. Second best sport: table tennis, in which she also represented Preston, and is playing again now.

St. Mary's College comment: She smoked heavily (some 50 cigarettes daily) until May last year, when she used hypnosis to help her give up altogether. Though carrying slightly more weight than the others, her flexibility was good, and she is quite strong. Her reaction time is only reasonable, but she demonstrated a by-no-means-bad endurance ability. If she trained harder and lost a little bit of weight, she is still young enough to do better.

TEST RESULTS. Height 5 ft ¼ in. Weight: 10 st 2 lb. RPI: 11·50. Grip strength: Right hand – 82 lb. Left hand – 77 lb. Flexibility: 16·5 cm. Simple reaction time 0·234 sec. Haemoglobin (g/100 m): 13·0. Vital capacity (litres): 3·55. FEV: 66%. Exercise heart rate (bpm): 145. VO2 (m/kg/min): 29·50. Smokes: No. Drinks alcohol: Yes.

Betty Condon. From Bickley, Kent, aged 55, widowed when 52, no children, working as a civil servant and caring for elderly parents. Four times British long-distance veteran champion, and current record-holder for the BLDSA's veterans championship, she swims an hour a day six days a week in summer, less in winter. Second best sport: netball, but has not played since 1967. She believes firmly that swimming affected her attitude to her bereavement, helped her to endure it and to face up to life again: 'It's a mental attitude that comes as an additional benefit.'

St. Mary's College comment: A remarkable example of how physical recreational activity can help somebody overcome life's traumas. She even had a major abdominal operation in 1970, and though she is not particularly strong, she competes at a high level of swimming in her own age group. Like all the other swimmers tested, she exudes an obvious enjoyment of life.

TEST RESULTS. Height: 5 ft 4½ in. Weight: 9 st 3 lb. RPI: 12·90. Grip strength: Right hand – 58 lb. Left hand – 49 lb. Flexibility: 19·0 cm. Simple reaction time 0·214 sec.

Haemoglobin (g/11 ml): 14·6. Vital capacity (litres): 3·08. FEV: 78·5%. Exercise heart rate (bpm): 165. VO2 (m/kg/min): 25·50. Smokes: No. Drinks alcohol: No.

Willy van Rysel. From Bournemouth, Hampshire, aged 61, married, no children, formerly worked as a commercial artist–designer. A highly successful long-distance swimmer, once a competition diver, now a renowned veteran swimmer who in 1977 returned from the USA National Short Course Masters Championship with five silver medals, and from the Long Course Masters Championships with three gold and two silver medals. She trains about three days a week, an hour on each occasion. Known for her spritely sense of humour. Second best sport: badminton, which she still plays.

St. Mary's College comment: Remarkably free from any history of illness. She's reasonably strong, reasonably flexible and has pretty good endurance. Can clearly elevate her heart rate to quite a high level, and maintain it there for some time. An advertisement for exercise.

TEST RESULTS. Height: 5 ft 4½ in. Weight: 10 st 4 lb. RPI: 12·15. Grip strength: Right hand – 73 lb. Left hand – 66 lb. Flexibility: 3·8 cm. Simple reaction time 0·210 sec. Haemoglobin (g/100 ml): 10·2. Vital capacity (litres): 2·75. FEV: 93%. Exercise heart rate (bpm): 150. VO2 (m/kg/min): 25·50. Smokes: No. Drinks alcohol: No.

Vivienne Cherriman. From Whitwell, Isle of Wight, aged 70, married, six children, working as a senior lecturer in law. An all-round sportswoman, particularly successful in swimming and diving competitions in the 1930s, she's now a long-distance swimmer who first swam from Ryde to Southsea in 1971, the first time it had been swum by a person over 60. Takes part in some physical activity every day, not necessarily swimming. Second best sport: table tennis, in which she was the English women's veteran champion in 1958. Nowadays she competes in golf as well as swimming events, and thinks nothing of playing golf in the morning, swimming in the afternoon and playing table tennis in the evening. She also jogs. Wishes she had been born later so that she could have played football.

St. Mary's College comment: An incredible person who has nothing really very much wrong with her. Her respiratory system is in good order. She is not very strong, but one would expect that. Nevertheless, she did well on the bicycle, working at a load many younger women would have been pleased to cope with. She bears out the fact that you can continue swimming at a high level to a ripe old age, particularly when the level of skill is high. Her reaction time was slow, and probably was, for some reason, not nearly as good as it is in a non-test situation. After all, following the tests, she beat another woman, more than 20 years her junior, at table tennis, and the other woman is a very good player!

TEST RESULTS. Height: 5 ft 2¼ in. Weight: 9 st 8 lb. RPI: 12·30. Grip strength: Right hand – 55 lb. Left hand – 61 lb. Flexibility: 14·0 cm. Simple reaction time 0·566 sec. Haemoglobin (g/100 ml): 13·3. Vital capacity (litres): 2·78. FEV: 93·5%. Exercise heart rate (bpm): 140. VO2 (m/kg/min): 32·00. Smokes: No. Drinks alcohol: Rarely.

MEN

James Stewart. From Westerham, Kent, aged 34, married, one child, working as an oil company executive. A top competitive swimmer in the early 1970s, he might have made the England team but for career commitments. He now swims for half an hour four days a week, has found like all the swimmers that the activity helps in controlling weight. After leaving school he put on two stones and then lost it in six months by swimming regularly. Moreover, as somebody who has suffered from asthma, he recommends swimming as a way also of alleviating, even curing, the condition. 'The breathing in swimming is like yoga breathing, which is also good for it.' Second best sport: rugby, which he still occasionally plays. Immediately before the tests, he was at a particularly low point (for him) physically, having worked three nights a week until two in the morning, for two successive weeks, preparing a report.

St. Mary's College comment: Had polio at the age of four, when he lost the use of muscles in both legs, principally the left, for a time, and was helped in his recovery by a physiotherapist aunt. Has also had a double hernia. He is a big man, quite strong, who gives the impression of being reasonably fit. His problem, clearly, is that like many men in their thirties, he is in the middle of the most critical part of his career and family life. If he can keep going now at a reasonable level, keeping fit later on will be all the easier. His regular swimming can only help in this.

TEST RESULTS. Height: 6 ft 2¼ in. Weight: 14 st 6 lb. RPI: 12·40. Grip strength: Right hand – 126 lb. Left hand – 116 lb. Flexibility: 7·6 cm. Simple reaction time 0·193 sec. Haemoglobin (g/100 ml): 16·0. Vital capacity (litres): 5·25. FEV: 84%. Exercise heart rate (bpm): 160. VO2 (m/kg/min): 36·00. Smokes: No. Drinks alcohol: In moderation.

Charles Doxat. From Weybridge, Surrey, aged 35, married, two children, a company director in an advertising agency. A former county swimming champion, he is president of the Otter Swimming Club, and swims three days a week for health reasons, 'to overcome business troubles, booze and Havana cigars', an hour on each occasion. Second best sport: running, which he no longer does.

St. Mary's College comment: Physically in pretty good shape, lively, energetic and works very hard, but clearly enjoys it. On the bicycle, he handled the same workload as some members of the national rowing squad.

TEST RESULTS. Height: 5 ft 11¼ in. Weight: 12 st 8 lb. RPI: 12·55. Grip strength: Right hand – 101 lb. Left hand – 95 lb. Flexibility: 6·4 cm. Simple reaction time 0·205 sec. Haemoglobin (g/100 ml): 14·0. Vital capacity (litres): 4·95. FEV: 90·5%. Exercise heart rate (bpm): 150. VO2 (m/kg/min): 45·20. Smokes: Two cigars a day. Drinks alcohol: Yes.

Dr. Roger Lloyd-Mostyn. From Mansfield, Nottingham-shire, aged 36, married, two children; a consultant physi-cian in a local hospital. Takes part in some physical activity about five days a week, if not swimming, then some form of hard manual work. Second best sport: cross-country running, though has not run seriously for some time.

St. Mary's College comment: Among the men, the slim-mest person tested, and for his size has a high vital lung capacity and a good forced expiratory volume. He is also above average in terms of strength, has good flexibility and, again taking into account his size, took quite a heavy workload on the stationary bicycle.

TEST RESULTS. Height: 5 ft 9½ in. Weight: 10 st 6 lb. RPI: 12·70. Grip strength: Right hand – 111 lb. Left hand – 110 lb. Flexibility: 7·6 cm. Simple reaction time 0·233 sec. Haemoglobin (g/100 ml): 14·6. Vital capacity (litres): 5·30. FEV: 97%. Exercise heart rate (bpm): 165. VO2 (m/kg/min): 35. Smokes: No. Drinks alcohol: Yes.

Robert Burn. From Beckenham, Kent, aged 40, two children; a company director of a printing firm. An ASA national team member in 1956, he now swims twice a week for pleasure, still plays club second-team water polo. Second best sport: golf, in which he competes nearly every week of the year.

St. Mary's College comment: Fitter than the average 40-year-old. A fairly big man, he has quite good flexibility and a good reaction time. He is maintaining a lot of his strength, and is still 'with it'.

TEST RESULTS. Height: 5 ft 9½ in. Weight: 13 st 8 lb. RPI: 12·10. Grip strength: Right hand – 146 lb. Left hand – 130 lb. Flexibility: 5·1 cm. Simple reaction time: 0·178 sec. Haemoglobin (g/100 ml): 15·2. Vital capacity (litres): 5·05. FEV: 98%. Exercise heart rate (bpm): 150. VO2 (m/kg/min): 40·60. Smokes: One to two cigars a day. Drinks alcohol: Yes.

John Lovesey. From Wandsworth, London, aged 45,

married, four children; newspaper sports editor. Swam for his school, took up swimming again on a regular basis in middle-age and now swims anything up to five times a week, for half an hour each time. Second best sport: cross-country running. Still runs for health reasons, anything up to six days a week.

St. Mary's College comment: Strong enough for what he wants to do, and particularly strong, relatively, in the lower body. Fit for his age, and able to train moderately hard.

TEST RESULTS. Height: 5 ft 7 in. Weight: 10 st 10 lb. RPI: 12·5. Grip strength: Right hand – 97 lb. Left hand – 93 lb. Flexibility: 9 cm. Simple reaction time 0·198 sec. Haemoglobin (g/100 ml): 14·6. Vital capacity (litres): 4·55. FEV: 97%. Exercise heart rate (bpm): 145. VO2 (m/kg/min): 44·00. Smokes: No. Drinks alcohol: Yes.

Douglas Payne. From Upminster, Essex, aged 47, married, two children; a bank manager. Swims only about once a week, but for two hours at a time, and also competes in thirty organised water polo competitions a year. Second best sport: running, which he no longer does.

St. Mary's College comment: No pun is intended but he is an example of somebody who has got something in the bank. He looks a typically middle-aged executive, a bit overweight, and he probably does not take enough exercise, but he scored better than expected. On the bicycle, he worked at a heavy load at a relatively low heart rate.

TEST RESULTS. Height: 5 ft 10¼ in. Weight: 14 st 3 lb. RPI: 12·10. Grip strength: Right hand – 117 lb. Left hand – 123 lb. Flexibility: 10·2 cm. Simple reaction time 0·200 sec. Haemoglobin (g/100 ml): 13·2. Vital capacity (litres): 4·85. FEV: 94%. Exercise heart rate (bpm): 145. VO2 (m/kg/min): 38·00. Smokes: Five cigars a day. Drinks alcohol: Yes.

Ron Roberts. From Bromley, Kent, aged 56, married, two children; an ex-police officer now working as a security executive. A former national record-holder in the

110 yards freestyle who swam for Britain in the Olympics at Helsinki and Melbourne, he was at his peak, unusually for a swimmer, at the age of 32. He still swims up to four times a week and can, with a build-up of training, get below a minute for 100 yards. 'Swimming,' he claims, 'is a lot better than any medicine I ever had.' Second best sport: cricket, but he does not play much now. Has the odd round of golf.

St. Mary's College comment: On the bicycle, he worked at a fairly high load and he is quite strong. He is not particularly flexible, but he is not overweight.

TEST RESULTS. Height: 5 ft 11½ in. Weight: 14 st 11 lb. RPI: 12·20. Grip strength: Right hand – 115 lb. Left hand – 115 lb. Flexibility: 1·3 cm. Simple reaction time 0·211 sec. Haemoglobin (g/100 ml): 13·8. Vital capacity (litres): 4·47. FEV: 74%. Exercise heart rate (bpm): 155. VO2 (m/kg/min): 22·50. Smokes: 2 cigars a week. Drinks alcohol: Yes.

Commander Gerald Forsberg. From Morecambe, Lancashire, aged 65, married, two grown-up children; a retired naval officer now working as an author and journalist. Renowned as a long-distance swimmer, he held the English Channel record from England to France from 1957 to 1959, and still swims six or seven days a week, covering a mile or more each time. He now competes in some ten distance events a year. Second best sport: was football.

St. Mary's College comment: He is close to being overweight, but he is a strong, even though a small man, who has lost some flexibility due to his prosperous-looking paunch. His reaction time would be acceptable from someone in their twenties. His lung capacity is not big, but he comes close to his capacity in forced expiratory volume, which indicates his muscles are in good trim. If he lost some weight Gerald Forsberg could probably push himself harder than he does, but he says he would greatly miss the protection of the fat layer during prolonged cold swims in the sea and lakes. He has told us to call him in 30 years' time for a follow-up study.

TEST RESULTS. Height: 5 ft 5¾ in. Weight: 13 st 11 lb. RPI: 11·40. Grip strength: Right hand – 97 lb. Left hand – 84 lb. Flexibility: minus 7·6 cm. Simple reaction time 0·205 sec. Haemoglobin (g/100 ml): 14·7. Vital capacity (litres): 3·20. FEV: 72%. Exercise heart rate (bpm): 150. VO2 (m/kg/min): 20. Smokes: Five half-coronas a day. Drinks alcohol: Yes.

The lesson to be learned

What emerged from the tests was a quite remarkable picture, proof of the value of swimming to health. Generally, the swimmers were free from illness, had undergone little major surgery and were strong. Most of them retained the reactions of 20-year-olds, and demonstrated an impressive cardio-vascular efficiency.

On the bicycle, they were able to sustain high workloads without undue stress. Mrs. Cherriman, for example, was able to pedal against a force that few women in their sixties would be able to manage, let alone at 70 like herself. Two of the men, Ron Roberts, 57, and Bob Burns, 40, kept pedalling at levels some members of the national rowing squad were working at later in the day. And if, in the area of physical ageing, muscular power is the first and fastest thing to deteriorate, Roberts and Burns could take heart from the fact that the following week two 16-year-old boys could not cope at all with the load they handled.

All the swimmers, as one might expect, were good, and sometimes excellent, in the business of expelling air from the lungs. And, in this connection, it is significant that within the group smoking was rare. If one of them smoked, the significance was minimal in terms of either the number of cigarettes smoked daily or the form, such as cigar smoking in which inhalation does not generally occur. The one person who had smoked considerably, fifty cigarettes a day, was one of three in the group who had suffered from bronchial asthma.

What is often raised about such examinations of selected groups of physically active individuals, is the proposition that healthy people have a predisposition towards sports

66

not shared by their less fortunate brethren. In other words, it is argued that it is not necessarily physical exercise that gives people good health. Rather that possessing good health makes people incline towards taking up sport. From this, the thought runs – among some doctors, scientists and statisticians – that you cannot conclude that running, jumping and playing games and swimming are the reasons why some people live longer, or lead lives that are relatively untroubled by illness. But it is an argument from which support is seeping steadily away, if only because the diseases brought about by bodily disuse are now so widespread, while the evidence in favour of exercise grows increasingly impressive.

A report published in April, 1977, by the Social Services and Employment Sub-Committee of the Expenditure Committee of the House of Commons, which has made a special inquiry into preventive medicine, emphasised this. It recommended that 'the relevant Government departments . . . should actively promote the practice of physical exercise, in a suitable form, for all age groups, as a positive contribution to preventive medicine. They should impress on everyone the need to take more physical exercise, even if this only means walking to work instead of using transport. Parents should encourage their children to walk to school where it is possible and safe to do so.'

In the previous year, the report of a joint working party of the Royal College of Physicians of London and the British Cardiac Society was similarly explicit. 'There is sufficient evidence,' it said, 'to justify a major concern about the sedentary life in relation to coronary heart disease, and to justify efforts to encourage the habit of physical activity at all ages and in both men and women. This seems reasonable and prudent, even though we have no definitive evidence regarding just how much physical activity or what degree of physical fitness is required to protect against coronary heart disease.'

Integral with all this is the increasing cost of the National Health Service – whatever its political hue, any Government is going, in future, to be concerned with that. As the

White Paper, Prevention and Health, published in December, 1977, pointed out, the high and increasing share of NHS expenditure is 'being devoted to the hospital services, most of which are curative services, compared with the relatively small sums spent on prevention'. Indeed, in 1976 the Central Council of Physical Recreation contended that it was costing the nation £300 million annually 'in dealing with the problems caused by lack of fitness resulting in some form of (related) heart disease'. It said that £20 million was being spent each year on tranquillisers alone.

The National Health Service has been in existence for three decades and the result was evaluated by Donald Gould in the *New Statesman*. 'During that time,' he wrote, 'Britons have been privileged to enjoy one of the most comprehensive and readily accessible systems of medical care in the world, served by doctors and nurses and other health workers trained to a pitch of excellence as high as may be found, and there have also been major advances in therapy. However, while the past decades *have* seen a dramatic change in the pattern of disease, there has been no reduction in the total incidence of ill health.'

The group of swimmers who took the tests at St. Mary's College can thus, at least, add a footnote to these pronouncements by their evident good health. Three cases are particularly relevant in relation to idea that it is people, untroubled by illness or physical affliction, who have a predilection for sporting activity. Firstly, Betty Condon, who had an operation many women might consider to be a major emotional calamity but who continued swimming for pleasure and furthermore, for competitive success. Secondly, James Stewart, who had polio as a child, suffered from asthma and has had a double hernia. And thirdly, Jean Chipperfield, with whom we began this book. She had suffered hepatitis, an extremely debilitating disease of the liver, and also frequent common colds, sore throats and tonsillitis. She then took up swimming and now has an Amateur Swimming Association teaching certificate. Her health improved out of all apparent proportion to the time spent in the pool.

CHAPTER EIGHT

Getting into the Swim

If the results of the St. Mary's College tests do not convince you of the value of swimming to your general good health, then I have to admit you are probably a lost cause. Nevertheless, if you are merely saying that you have not got the time to exercise, then I will respond with the reply of one of those who featured in the series on middle-age fitness in the *Sunday Times*: 'If you haven't got time to exercise, then you'll have to find time to be ill.'

Dr. Leo Walkden, who is the honorary doctor to the British Long Distance Swimming Association and the Rugby Football Union is a long-distance swimmer and jogger himself. He had those words up in big type in his surgery until somebody pinched them. Dr. Walkden was present at the tests on 70-year-old Mrs. Cherriman and her fellow swimmers and if, like him, you are impressed, what follows in the next chapter are a series of training schedules which will help you comfortably to build up fitness in the pool, and proceed to a competent competitive level if you wish.

The schedules are provided by Hamilton Smith, coach to the English national team 1963–67 and to the Scottish national team 1969–70, now the executive director of the British Swimming Coaches' Association, whose book *Learning to Swim and Dive* (published by Collins) is one I would recommend to anyone who is either teaching himself to swim, or teaching others.

Depending on your degree of ability and assuming you have no coach, you will at some time need to purchase a book on technique since this book is not technical, nor does it assume an inability to swim on the part of the reader.

The problem for most of us is to translate swimming

69

ability into an interesting and progressive exercise schedule. Until I met Hamilton Smith, a Scot with a briskness of manner that fails to hide his basic belief in sport as something enjoyable, I was a swimmer who ploughed endlessly up and down a pool, using one stroke almost exclusively. The discipline this required was not to be sneered at, but I often felt in agreement with people who said they found such unrelenting training on a single stroke simply boring. You can think about other things, even solve problems, while swimming in this way but it can often prove monotonous, to say the least.

Hamilton Smith brought the fun back into swimming for me, and I believe his schedules can create a great deal of joy for other swimmers of whatever standard. The schedules are not only novel; more important, they are a recommendation for swimming as one of the best, if not *the* best, exercise activity for any age. They are not, crucially, broken into age groups, but into levels in which swimming skill and experience are the important criteria, rather than age or physical condition.

Although nobody can afford to ignore those last two factors, the nature of swimming is such, as Hamilton Smith says, that with steady all-round limb movements done with the body completely supported by water, age and physical condition have much less effect on the training routine than they have on land-based activities. An out-of-shape man or woman who goes running, for example, can end up extremely stiff the following day, but whoever heard of that happening to a swimmer except somebody – like a champion – who knew how to push really hard?

Whatever your age, the schedules meet the needs of all sorts of people, ranging from those who have overcome the first problems of learning to swim, but who have not developed any stroke technique, to those with a background of swimming at club or school.

In following them, it is to be emphasised strongly that the body *adapts* to exercise, and if it is to do this properly, there must be a gradual increase in the intensity of the sessions. Fail to observe this, and your body will react; it will object, and physical and psychological harm can result. This is easy to understand if you imagine, as an extreme case, what could happen to a man who attempted to run a marathon having never run farther than 800 yards before in his life.

So progress at your own rate, training not straining, and you will discover that though there are times when you do not go forward at all, there will also be gains which will bring a lift like few others you will ever experience. Improvement can be a matter of months rather than days, but even people in their sixties and seventies once fit, can look forward to managing easily half a mile or more eventually. The water then seems to sing in your ears.

As you may have already concluded, the best plan is to swim regularly. This is more important than trying to attempt a frequency that you know you may never keep up. The aim is, after all, a long-term one directed towards enjoyment and fitness from swimming, rather than a more immediate goal of a top-class performance in a race. Even so, if you are serious, you should be willing to swim at least twice a week. Three or four times a week would be even better. Try to build up a schedule that means you are in the pool when it is likely to be less populated with other swimmers; early morning is often the best time, but conditions vary according to locality and time of year.

The schedules, with their emphasis on all-round ability and variety, will tend to get you more easily through the plateau periods, when no progress seems to be made. But if you have only one stroke – breaststroke for instance – do not despair. The level at which the schedules start is designed to help you master other strokes, and if you feel either front or back crawl or butterfly is beyond you, consider mastering something simple like sidestroke or elementary backstroke. The sidestroke is illustrated on page 73 and the elementary backstroke on page 76; in the intervening two pages the four competitive strokes are displayed.

Both the sidestroke and elementary backstroke are easy strokes, which can let you rest and yet still allow you to make headway through the water. If you know how to do the sidestroke, which was a competitive stroke three-quarters of a century ago, you can rescue somebody in the water because the side position enables you to carry the victim or rescue equipment. In both these strokes, you can breathe naturally, in and out through the mouth.

A variation of the elementary backstroke is the inverted breaststroke. The difference is that the timing of the kick and arms is alternated. It is worth trying if only to test the efficiency of your breaststroke kick.

In looking at the schedules, particularly if you are older, be honest with yourself. 'It is better,' according to Hamilton Smith, 'to start at a lower level and work upwards rather than be put off, first by discomfort and secondly by dismay at failing to meet your target.' If in any doubt at all, it is a good idea to spend a few sessions trying out some of the schedules and assessing yourself that way. Nobody will know better than you what you are ready for.

Generally speaking, there are two kinds of errors that affect a swimmer's efficiency: those that increase resistance in the water unnecessarily, and those that use energy without contributing sufficient propulsive power. There are several points worth pondering that will pay dividends if you have not been swimming regularly before starting on one of the schedules, or even if you have. So remember:

One, try to relax. If you screw up your face or keep your eyes too tightly shut tension will be created in other parts of the body. This will not only restrict your efficiency, but tire you very quickly. If you drive a car, you may recall how tired you felt when you first started, because you failed to relax. The same thing can happen in the water.

Two, the water is a cushion. Most people with their lungs partially inflated are slightly buoyant, and lighter than water, so will float at the surface. However, a human being is not a duck but more like a dog, which swims with only a small part of itself out of the water. As you go faster, the body will rise slightly due to the resistance it encounters on the underneath part. That is why it is important to keep the head in line with the body to give a streamline effect; the

SIDESTROKE

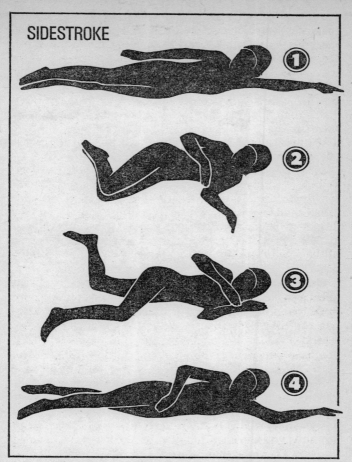

1. In the glide, the top arm is at the side, the bottom arm outstretched with the palm down, and the legs are together with toes pointed.

2. The bottom arm is pressed down through the water, delivering its power first, until the fingers point to the bottom. Then the two arms go into the recovery phase, both hands being brought to the bottom shoulder as the knees are bent.

3. The legs are spread in a wide V.

4. As the top arm is now pressed down and back across to the body's side, simultaneously the legs are whipped together while the bottom arm completes the recovery to its original position (1).

FRONT CRAWL

BACK CRAWL

BREAST STROKE

BUTTERFLY

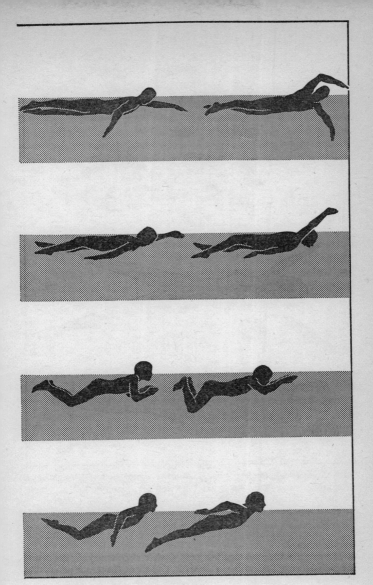

ELEMENTARY BACKSTROKE

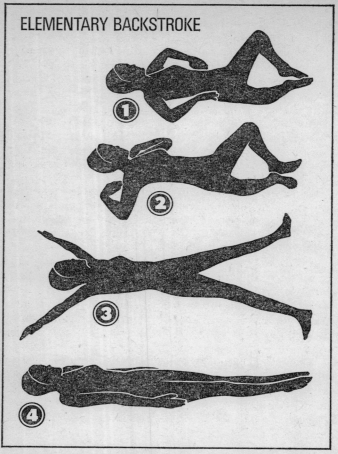

1. In the recovery, the knees are bent outward and the legs brought into a diamond shape, the elbows are bent and the hands moved up along the body.

2. From this position the wrists are turned outward. Remember that the arms stay in the water throughout the stroke.

3. As the legs are slowly spread apart in a wide V, the arms extend full length outward.

4. The legs are whipped together gently, while simultaneously the arms are pulled through the water to the sides. Exhale on the stroke and make the glide last two or three seconds. Inhale on the recovery (1).

Drawings by John Grimwade

back should never be arched, and you should not try to 'climb' on top of the water.

Three, in the water, arm and leg movements are much more carefully controlled and less dynamic than on land. To gain maximum propulsion you should not try to 'tear a hole' in the water with the hands and feet, but aim for a full range of continuous, long, firm movements with each stroke. Underwater shots of great swimmers have demonstrated that they create far fewer bubbles below the surface than inferior performers. Try to emulate them – not the noisy, splashy person trying in the summer sun to make an impression on friends.

Four, if you pull powerfully enough you can feel effort in the water. One reason some recreational swimmers never progress is that swimming is an activity in which the shoulder and arm muscles, in particular, can provide proof of effort. The feeling can be the same as that given by a series of press-ups on land – a pleasant muscular ache. If you fail to work hard, you will never experience this, and will not improve.

Five, breathing in a pool needs to be controlled. If you place your head under water, the pressure outside your nose and mouth is greater than the pressure inside. As a result, water enters the mouth and nose and, in the case of the beginner, can choke him. Closing your mouth when your head is under water and exhaling a small amount of air constantly through your nose, is a good way to prevent this happening. By the time you are completely accustomed to the water, you will be balancing the pressure inside your nose and mouth so that it is equal to the pressure outside and no water will enter. You will also be blowing out, partly into the water as bubbles and partly into the air as an explosive pant, and inhaling when the mouth is well clear of the water, thus avoiding unpleasant swallowing. Be aware that if breathing is a problem, you must be patient. As you become fitter and more skilled and therefore more relaxed, a proper pattern of breathing will emerge quite naturally until one day you will wonder what all the worry was about. If necessary, practise blowing the air out hard and rhythmically with your face below the surface.

Six, keep your eyes open both above and below the water.
They will automatically and instinctively close as they pass
through the actual water surface. You can, of course, wear
goggles, which are discussed in this book. Nevertheless, if
you are not at ease in the water, it will help for a time to
adjust to this slight discomfort until, like breathing, you
hardly give it a thought. It's part of the learning process.

**Seven, your balance is disorientated by your horizontal
position.** Thus, do not make exaggerated compensatory
movements simply because you are not vertical.

**Eight, always allow time for your body to adjust to the
water.** Anyone who has swum in the sea will know that the
hardest part often is getting into the water – simply over-
coming the reluctance to face the inevitable shock of water
on warm skin. This will occur no matter how warm the
water is. It can be an exhilarating experience for many, but
not all. I remember watching Bobby McGregor, who won
the silver medal in the Olympic 100 metres freestyle in
1964, training before Tokyo. His period of adjustment gave
me the start to a story in *Sports Illustrated*:

'If there is one thing Bobby McGregor hates, it is swimming first thing in the morning. Bobby is a tall, lithe 20-
year-old Scot, and one of the fastest swimmers in history.
He is also one of the most reluctant, which may account
for the fact that he is solid favourite for the 100 metres
freestyle gold medal in the Tokyo Olympics at an age when
many top swimmers are burned out. Bobby approaches his
daily 7.30 a.m. workout with deep revulsion. He walks into
the pool at the shallow end, shuddering. His chest is puffed
out, and he tiptoes slowly forward, delaying the moment of
total immersion as long as possible.'

You can help to overcome the sort of shock Bobby Mc-
Gregor so hated by jumping and splashing about a bit. You
should then orientate yourself to the horizontal position –
practising turns is a useful part of this process. Do turns
with the minimum amount of fuss, but remember that a
good, strong push-off will be valuable in maintaining
momentum and rhythm.

After a warm-up, to complete the conquering of what we can call the 'McGregor phase', the emphasis of each set of schedules is on:

1. Continuous swims. In which the distance covered will be gradually increased.
2. Interval swims. In which you will swim a set distance several times with rest periods carefully built in.
3. Challenge swims. In which you will, if ready, move forward quite significantly.

Nevertheless, the schedules are not hard-and-fast regimens which you cannot vary or break. They are essentially a guide which you should follow at your discretion. For example, where a rest period is not mentioned, you can rest between drills to complete recovery (i.e. until you are breathing normally), and you should always rest to complete recovery after a key swim.

The emphasis on a variety of strokes is intended to make for a mixture of stresses. The different strokes not only exercise different muscles, but allow you to continue swimming longer, when you are fatigued on one stroke, you go on with another.

You will notice that some of the drills require a kickboard. Later in the book, I provide some details which will help you obtain the right types. The technique employed with them is simple: When you are using a board for leg-kicking practice, you hold the board near the top, with the fingers underneath and the thumbs on top. You keep your head up so that breathing can take place easily, while you concentrate on the leg action. For leg-kicking practise on the back, you hold the board flat to the chest, gripping it in the same way, but in the middle with the elbows to the side, and the top under the chin. If you do want to use a board for armstroke practice, and find it difficult to simply let the legs trail, then a large kickboard is unsuitable, and you need a small one which you grip between the top of the thighs. There is also on the market equipment specially designed to hold the legs in the swimming position, while doing arms-only practice, and details of this, I also cover later.

Do not train too soon after eating. It will certainly be uncomfortable and if you are going to swim vigorously I would suggest putting no less than two hours between your session and the immediately previous meal.

Training, not straining, is emphasised even in the schedules' challenge swims which, in the first few levels, merely increase the distance of continuous swims. Later on, the challenge swims switch to tests of time and distance, so providing some extra objectivity. You can better measure your improvement, and ensure the overload necessary to progress.

Remember, just as a runner, after a period of strenuous exertion does not stop entirely, neither should a swimmer. Therefore get into the habit after each session, whether it has concentrated on skill development or training for distance and time, of enjoying a few moments of relaxation, experimenting or just having fun in the water. It will help to restore the body's equilibrium, and this is important.

When deciding where you fit best into Hamilton Smith's conditioning courses, bear in mind that if you are over 35 and have any doubts at all about your fitness or have had a serious illness, you should first seek the clearance of your doctor. Then, whatever schedule you choose, you should start gradually and repeat each session within it until you can handle it comfortably. Never move from one session to the next, or change schedules, before you are sure you can cope.

How you feel will be your best guide and in judging your fitness to move on, you will find it helpful to keep a diary of the details of each session, with comments on your own reactions. You could also include other details, like your weight and pulse rate, taken each morning, and thus derive a sense of satisfaction from your progress all round, particularly when you look back. Crucially, a diary will help you to know yourself better. Every individual is different, and while care has been taken to cater in the schedules for a wide range, in the end you may need to plan your own sessions.

CHAPTER NINE

The Training Schedules

At the beginning of each set of Hamilton Smith's schedules is a description of swimming-ability level. These will help you to decide where to start. The schedules assume a pool-length of approximately 25 metres. Where it is not possible to swim widths as indicated, use half-lengths. Other adjustments will be necessary for different lengths of pool. Now choose a schedule, and *start straight away*.

THE BEGINNER. This person is able to swim, and is fairly happy in the water, but has no real experience in any of the strokes. The programme is therefore based on stroke development, working mainly on widths and concentrating on a good stretch and streamlined body position, with the face in the water and the eyes open, and pushing from the poolside and gliding; regular breathing, blowing out bubbles into the water before exhaling into the air, and proper stroke patterns, using the whole-stroke and part-stroke drills and practices. At this level, particularly, the sessions are examples of what you may do. There is no need to follow them slavishly. Have fun.

Session 1

Warm-up. Accustom to temperature by walking, jumping, splashing. Completely immerse. Try flotation practices, curled up and stretched on both the back and the front. Push and glide towards and away from poolside. Practise breathing, blow bubbles into water

Skill development: 1st choice stroke
2 widths – full stroke
2 widths – legs only (use kickboard)
2 widths – arms only (use kickboard)
2 widths – full stroke, concentrating primarily on
          breathing
2 widths – full stroke

Skill development: 2nd choice stroke
Same schedule as 1st choice stroke

Easy swim. Fun and games, diving, blowing bubbles, etc.

Session 2	As for Session 1 but use 1st choice stroke and 3rd choice stroke
Session 3	1st and 2nd choice stroke
	Warm-up. As for Session 1
	Skill development. Same practices as Session 1 but do 4 widths on each section.
	Easy swim. As for Session 1
Session 4	As for Session 3, but use 1st choice stroke and 3rd choice stroke
Session 5	Same pattern as previously, but work on all 3 strokes
CHALLENGE	**Warm-up.** As in Session 1
	Skill development. Swim as many widths on 1st choice stroke as possible without overdue fatigue or excessive loss of good technique

THE CONVERT. In this case we have somebody who is hooked, but who is still able to swim only a short distance – perhaps one length, using a recognisable but not very efficient stroke. The programme is therefore based on a careful combination of stroke development as for the previous level, but with a gradual build-up of distance while trying to maintain the correct stroke patterns. In following the programme, if one stroke is done more efficiently, or feels better than the others, use it more than the others, though do not neglect them. The ultimate aim, remember, is to achieve an all-round skill improvement. Try for smooth strokes and a full, regular breathing pattern. And practise an easy turning movement. Enjoy yourself.

Session 1	**Warm-up.** As for Beginner's Session 1, plus single widths $\times 2$ on each stroke, thinking of technical points and aiming for steady stroke rate. Try turning practice on 1st choice stroke
	Skill development
	1 length 1st choice stroke – rest to recovery
	Repeat above
	4 widths – 2nd choice stroke
	4 widths – 3rd choice stroke
	Build up the number of widths as you wish
	Easy swim. Experiment with flotation and fun.
	This session should be repeated until you are ready for more lengths on 1st choice stroke and/or 1 length on 2nd or 3rd choice stroke

Session 2	**Warm-up.** As for Session 1

Skill development
1 length – 1st choice stroke
Repeat above
1 length – 2nd choice stroke
1 length – 1st choice stroke
Widths – 2 or more on each stroke. Revise technique

Easy swim

Repeat this session until you are able to complete each length in reasonable comfort, and breathing returns to normal fairly soon (about one minute)

Session 3	**Warm-up.** As for Session 1

Skill development
1 length – 1st choice stroke
1 length – 2nd choice stroke
2 lengths – 1st choice stroke
Aim for 1 minute rest between each length
6 or more widths – 2nd and 3rd choice strokes

Easy swim

Repeat this session until you can complete 2 lengths 1st choice stroke in reasonable comfort

Session 4	**Warm-up.** As for Session 1

Skill development
1 length – 1st choice stroke
1 length – 2nd choice stroke
2 lengths – 1st choice stroke
1 length – 3rd choice stroke
2 lengths – 1st choice stroke
1 length – 2nd choice stroke
Aim for 1 minute rest between lengths

Easy swim

This session should be repeated until each section is done with relative ease, with 1 minute maximum rest between each

Session 5	**Warm-up.** Vary slightly and cut to 4–5 minutes

Skill development
1 length – 1st choice stroke
1 length – 2nd choice stroke
1 length – 3rd choice stroke
3 lengths – 1st choice stroke
1 length – 2nd choice stroke
1 length – 3rd choice stroke
2 lengths – 1st choice stroke

Easy swim

When this session can be completed without undue discomfort, you are now ready for a challenge swim

CHALLENGE	**Warm-up.** Fairly short adjustment practice on widths. Then 2 widths on each stroke

83

Challenge swim
1 length – 1st choice stroke
1 length – 2nd choice stroke
1 length – 3rd choice stroke
Swim as many lengths 1st choice stroke as possible in a maximum time of 15 minutes or less if preferred. Aim to keep stroke smooth and fairly efficient

Easy swim. Relaxation
After this swim you will be able to reassess your status, and should now move on to a new level. Choose carefully

THE TYRO. An interesting stage. One in which the swimmer can manage a reasonable distance on one or two strokes, but only when the face is kept clear of the water and breathing is unrestricted. This swimmer, in fact, tends to be unsure about putting the face in the water, and the programme is based on a combination of increasing fitness by doing some distance swims and gradually improving stroke technique. If you have among your strokes the front crawl, or have managed at least to master the rudiments of it, that is the one to concentrate on now in terms of skill, practising the legs and arms separately and gradually progressing from widths to lengths. If you have not got front crawl, this is the stage, provided you are swimming reasonable distances on another stroke, to try it. It can be the most satisfying stroke of all, and you may surprise yourself and your friends when you discover how easy it is. If necessary, get an instructor to advise you. And remember – be happy and relaxed in the water.

Session 1 **Warm-up.** Adjustment and orientation practices, including:
Flotation – try to lie flat and let the water hold you up.
Push and glide – towards and away from the wall, keeping face in the water, eyes open
Breathing practices – blow bubbles steadily into the water, lift head, take another breath and repeat rhythmically. Remember to relax the chest and face to eliminate tension

Skill development. Practise on single widths doing all three strokes. Try to keep the head in line with the body, and when your face is in the water keep your eyes open and breathe out as in the warm-up practice

Main training section
2 widths – 1st choice stroke
2 widths – 2nd choice stroke

1 width – Front crawl
Repeat this pattern a number of times

Easy swim. Relax and have fun

Session 2 **Warm-up.** A few minutes spent on adjustment and orientation, floating in curled and stretched positions. Pushing and gliding on front, face in water, eyes open, blowing bubbles into water and inhaling in a rhythmic way. 4 widths or 1 length on 1st choice stroke

Skill development: front crawl
2 widths – full stroke
2 widths – kicking, hands extended in front, face in water, eyes open
2 widths – single arm practice – i.e., hold one arm out in front, use other arm only. Alternate arms on widths
2 widths – full stroke without breathing
2 widths – full stroke, regular breathing

Main training section
1 length – 1st choice stroke
1 length – 2nd choice stroke
1 length – 1st choice stroke
1 length – 2nd choice stroke
Concentrate here on steady, smooth strokes and rest to recovery between each length

Easy swim

Repeat this session until able to complete without discomfort

Session 3 **Warm-up.** A few minutes adjustment – orientation as in Session 2. Then:
4 widths or 1 length – 1st choice stroke

Skill development: front crawl
3 widths – full stroke
2 widths – kicking, hands extended in front, face in water, eyes open
2 widths – kicking (use kickboard)
2 widths – full stroke
2 widths – single arm practice
2 widths – full stroke, without breathing
2 widths – full stroke, regular breathing

Main training section
1 length – 1st choice stroke
1 length – 2nd choice stroke
2 lengths – 1st choice stroke
1 length – 2nd choice stroke
1 length – 1st choice stroke
Aim to cut down rest to around 1 minute. Rest to recovery before 2 length swim

Easy swim. Practise turning

Repeat this until able to do 2 lengths 1st choice stroke with relative ease

Session 4	**Warm-up.** As for Session 3

Skill development: front crawl
4 widths – full stroke
2 widths – kicking, hands extended in front, face in
               water, eyes open
2 widths – kicking (use kickboard)
2 widths – full stroke
2 widths – single arm practice
2 widths – full stroke, without breathing
4 widths – full stroke, regular breathing

Main training section
1 length   – 1st choice stroke
1 length   – 2nd choice stroke
2 lengths – 1st choice stroke
2 lengths – 2nd choice stroke
1 length   – 1st choice stroke
1 length   – 2nd choice stroke
Aim for 1 minute rest between

Easy swim. Relax, practise dives and turns.
Repeat this until able to do 2 lengths on 1st and 2nd
choice strokes without discomfort

Session 5	**Warm-up.** As for Session 3

Skill development: front crawl
4 widths – full stroke
2 widths – kicking, hands extended in front, face in
               water, eyes open
2 widths – kicking (use kickboard)
4 widths – full stroke, but concentrating on pushing off
               and getting kick going before adding arms
2 widths – single arm practice
2 widths – catch-up stroke, i.e. pushing off with arms
               extended, as in single arm practice, and then
               alternate right and left arm strokes, ensuring
               that each arm extends in front alongside
               other before commencing next stroke
4 widths – full stroke, alternating 1 without breathing
               and 1 with regular breathing

Main training section
1 length   – 1st choice stroke
1 length   – 2nd choice stroke
2 lengths – 1st choice stroke
2 lengths – 2nd choice stroke
1 length   – 1st choice stroke
1 length   – 2nd choice stroke
1 length   – front crawl, holding steady stroke and
               breathing regularly. Stop if you need to hold
               your breath
1 length   – 1st choice stroke
Aim for 1 minute between swims, except before 1 length
front crawl – when rest to recover

Easy swim

Repeat until able to do full length on front crawl with ease

Session 6   **Warm-up.** As for Session 3

Skill development: all strokes

4 widths – front crawl, regular breathing
4 widths – 1st choice stroke
4 widths – 2nd choice stroke
4 widths – kicking (use kickboard)
Alternate widths front crawl with best other stroke
4 widths – alternate widths single-arm and catch-up practice on front crawl
4 widths – front crawl

Main training section

1 length – 1st choice stroke
1 length – front crawl
1 length – 2nd choice stroke
2 lengths – 1st choice stroke
1 length – front crawl
2 lengths – 2nd choice stroke
1 length – front crawl
1 length – 1st choice stroke
Aim to rest a maximum of 1 minute between each swim

Easy swim. Practise turns and relax.
Repeat until able to do each length on front crawl with no difficulties

Session 7   **Warm-up.** As for Session 3, but spend less time on it

Skill development

1 length – 1st choice stroke
1 length – front crawl
1 length – 2nd choice stroke
1 length – front crawl
Aim to perform strokes slowly and correctly, concentrating on distance per stroke and good breathing pattern

Main training section

1 length – 1st choice stroke
2 lengths – 2nd choice stroke
1 length – front crawl
3 lengths – 1st choice stroke
1 length – 2nd choice stroke
1 length – front crawl
1 length – 1st choice stroke
Aim to cut rest between each swim to maximum of 1 minute

Easy swim. Turning practice and relax.
Repeat until able to do each section with ease and with a fairly short rest. You are now ready to attempt a challenge swim

CHALLENGE   **Warm-up.** A few gentle widths on each stroke, concentrating on correct stroke patterns and regular breathing

Challenge swim
1 length – 1st choice stroke
1 length – front crawl (optional)
1 length – 2nd choice stroke
Swim as many lengths on 1st choice or a mixture of 1st and 2nd choice strokes, without stopping and at as steady a pace as possible, in 10 or 15 minutes. Note distance covered and record

Easy swim. Relax and have fun.
When you have completed this session you should be able to assess your present status and determine your next level and series of sessions

THE INITIATE. At this point, the swimmer is *really* enrolled. He is able to swim two strokes, back crawl and breaststroke reasonably competently. What's more, he can make a moderate attempt at front crawl, although only over a short distance, say a length, probably because of breathing difficulties. At this level, it is probably the most common class. An alternative but similar level of ability is epitomised in those able to swim front crawl and back crawl fairly competently, but unable to manage even a reasonable breaststroke. If you fall in this category, you can still use the following schedules but should spend some time on the breaststroke, utilising the sessions for the Beginner or Convert. Generally, the following sessions are based on a combination of distance build-up on two strokes with a gradual increase in the third-choice stroke, emphasising technique. An occasional session working almost exclusively on skill should be done. Keep smiling.

Session 1

Warm-up and skill practice. Short adjustment and orientation practice as described in Session 2 of the Tyro's schedule. Do only a few widths and practices

Skill development
1 length – 1st choice stroke
1 length – 2nd choice stroke
1 length – 3rd choice stroke
1 length – 1st choice stroke
Rest to recovery between each length, and concentrate on doing each stroke, on each length, as correctly and effectively as possible

Main training section
1 length – 1st choice stroke
1 length – 2nd choice stroke
1 length – 3rd choice stroke

88

1 length – 1st choice stroke
Rest until breathing is steady and fairly comfortable between swims

Easy swim. Practise turns and relax.
Repeat this session until you are able to finish each length in reasonable comfort

Session 2

Warm-up and skill practice. As for Session 1

Main training section
1 length – 1st choice stroke
1 length – 2nd choice stroke
1 length – 3rd choice stroke
2 lengths – 1st choice stroke
1 length – 2nd choice stroke
1 length – 3rd choice stroke
1 length – 1st choice stroke
Rest until breathing is steady and fairly comfortable between swims, and check the time taken to achieve this

Easy swim. Practise turns and relax.
Repeat until each swim can be done comfortably, especially the two lengths. You will find yourself gradually cutting down on rest time

Session 3

Warm-up and skill practice. As for Session 1

Main training section
1 length – 1st choice stroke
1 length – 2nd choice stroke
1 length – 3rd choice stroke
3 lengths – 1st choice stroke
2 lengths – 2nd choice stroke
1 length – 3rd choice stroke
1 length – 1st choice stroke
Rest for a maximum of 1 minute between swims, except before and after 3 lengths, when rest to recovery

Easy swim. Turns and relax

Repeat until able to hold stroke over each distance without discomfort

Session 4

Warm-up and skill practice. As for Session 1

Main training section
1 length – 1st choice stroke
2 lengths – 1st choice stroke
1 length – 2nd choice stroke
2 lengths – 2nd choice stroke
1 length – 3rd choice stroke
1 length – 3rd choice stroke
2 lengths – 2nd choice stroke
2 lengths – 1st choice stroke
Rest for 1 minute before 2 length swims, and less between others. Check this rest time on a clock

Easy swim. Practise turns and relax

Repeat until able to perform with no real discomfort during or after swims and rest is cut down

Session 5   **Warm-up and skill practice.** Brief orientation phase, swimming gently and concentrating on smooth stroke and regular breathing. Plus:
2 lengths – 1st choice stroke
1 length – 2nd choice stroke
1 length – 3rd choice stroke

Main training section
2 lengths – alternate lengths 1st and 2nd choice strokes
2 × 1 length – 3rd choice stroke
3 lengths – 1st choice stroke
2 lengths – 2nd choice stroke
2 × 1 length – 3rd choice stroke
2 lengths – alternate lengths 1st and 2nd choice strokes
1 length – 1st choice stroke, checking stroke count
Rest less than 1 minute between swims except after 3 lengths when rest to recovery

Easy swim. Practise turns and relax

Repeat until able to complete all swims in comfort, while resting as indicated

Session 6   **Warm-up and skill practice.** As for Session 5

Main training section
2 lengths – 1st choice stroke
       Rest 30–45 secs
2 lengths – alternate lengths 2nd and 3rd choice strokes
       Rest to recovery
4 lengths – 1st choice stroke
       Rest maximum 1 minute
2 × 1 length – 3rd choice stroke
       Rest maximum 1 minute between each length
3 lengths – 2nd choice stroke
       Rest maximum 1 minute
1 length – 3rd choice stroke
       Rest maximum 1 minute
1 length – 2nd choice stroke
       Rest maximum 1 minute
1 length – 1st choice stroke

Easy swim. Relax and have fun

This session may now be done alternating with Session 7

Session 7   **Warm-up.** – As for Session 5

Main training section
2 × 2 lengths – 1st choice stroke
Rest 30–45 secs between each 2 lengths
2 lengths – 2nd choice stroke
Rest maximum 1 minute

4 lengths – 1st choice stroke
Rest maximum 1 minute
2 lengths – 2nd choice stroke
Rest 30–45 secs
2 × 2 lengths – 1st choice stroke
Rest 30–45 secs between each 2 lengths

Easy swim.
This session may be done alternating with Session 6

Session 8   **Warm-up.** As for Session 5

Main training section
4 lengths – alternate lengths 1st and 2nd choice stroke
Rest maximum 1 minute
2 lengths – 3rd choice stroke
Rest maximum 1 minute
6 lengths – 1st choice stroke
Rest to recovery
2 lengths – 3rd choice stroke
Rest maximum 1 minute
4 lengths – Alternate lengths 1st and 2nd choice

Easy swim.
When this session can be done without difficulty with rests taken as indicated, you are ready for a challenge swim. This may be one of the following:

CHALLENGE 1   **Warm-up.** A few widths or lengths swimming gently and concentrating on correct stroke patterns, careful breathing and steady rhythms

Challenge swim
1 length – 1st choice stroke
1 length – 2nd choice stroke
1 length – 3rd choice stroke
1 length – 1st choice stroke
Rest until breathing is relaxed and steady

Swim non-stop for 15 minutes. Count the number of lengths covered to the nearest half-length and record. You may change strokes as you wish

Easy swim.
This session will be a good test of basic swimming endurance. Compare your results with:

CHALLENGE 2   **Warm-up.** As for Challenge 1

Main training section
1 length – 1st choice stroke
1 length – 2nd choice stroke
1 length – 3rd choice stroke
1 length – 1st choice stroke

Swim non-stop for 3 × 5 minutes with 1 minute rest between each swim

AND/OR

Swim non-stop for 5 × 3 minutes with 30 secs rest between each swim

91

Do not try to go fast at the start and aim for a steady continuous pace. Count the number of lengths covered to the nearest half-length and compare with Challenge 1

Easy swim. Relax

THE NOVICE. This is somebody who is able to swim three strokes with basically sound movement patterns, but who has never swum more than one or two lengths. The following schedule is thus based on a steady increase in endurance. The distances are increased, along with repetition swims. After a sound distance ability has been developed, time distance swims are introduced.

Session 1	**Warm-up.** A few minutes on adjustment practices. Flotation. Pushing and gliding from poolside stressing streamlining and breathing practices. Some widths on steady mixed-stroke swimming. Concentrate on precise stroke movements

Main training section
1 length – 1st choice stroke
1 length – 2nd choice stroke
1 length – 3rd choice stroke
1 length – 1st choice stroke
Rest to recovery before each length

Easy swim. Practise turns

Repeat this session a couple of times till able to complete each length without discomfort, and with reasonable stroke technique maintained throughout

Session 2	**Warm-up.** Remember to start gently with steady rhythmic strokes and breathing. Swim:

1 length – 1st choice stroke
1 length – 2nd choice stroke
1 length – 3rd choice stroke
1 length – 1st choice stroke
Attempt to keep the rest between each length to a maximum of 1 minute

Main training section
1 length – 1st choice stroke
1 length – 2nd choice stroke
1 length – 3rd choice stroke
1 length – 1st choice stroke
Aim for maximum of 1 minute rest between swims, but try to cut this down gradually

Easy swim. Practise turns

Repeat this session, aiming to cut down the rest between swims, but try to hold a good stroke

Session 3	**Warm-up.** As for Session 2

Warm-up. As for Session 2

Main training section
1 length – 1st choice stroke
1 length – 2nd choice stroke
1 length – 1st choice stroke
1 length – 3rd choice stroke
2 lengths – 1st choice stroke
Aim for a maximum of 50 secs rest between swims, except before the 2 lengths when rest to recovery

Easy swim. Relax and practise turns

Repeat this session until the rest is cut down, and you can do the 2 lengths without difficulty

Session 4

Warm-up. As for Session 2

Main training section
2 lengths – 1st choice stroke
1 length – 2nd choice stroke
1 length – 1st choice stroke
1 length – 3rd choice stroke
2 lengths – 1st choice stroke
Aim for maximum of 40 secs rest between swims

Easy swim.
Repeat this until the rest period is down to 30 secs between each swim

Session 5

Warm-up. As for Session 2

Main training section
2 lengths – 1st choice stroke
1 length – 2nd choice stroke
2 lengths – 1st choice stroke
1 length – 3rd choice stroke
3 lengths – 1st choice stroke
Aim for maximum of 30 secs rest between swims, except before 3 lengths when rest to recovery

Easy swim

Repeat until able to complete with rest and hold 3 lengths without difficulty

Session 6

Warm-up. Swim 4 lengths any strokes, any order. Hold a steady pace and rest as required, especially if breathing becomes stressed

Main training section
3 lengths – 1st choice stroke
1 length – 2nd choice stroke
3 lengths – 1st choice stroke
1 length – 3rd choice stroke
4 lengths – 1st choice stroke
Aim for a maximum of 30 secs rest between swims, except before 4 lengths when rest to recovery

Easy swim. Relax

Repeat until able to complete without undue strain,

keeping the rest periods down and you are capable of finishing 4 lengths fairly easily. You are now ready for some challenge swims

CHALLENGE **Warm-up.** Swim 4 lengths steady and rest to recovery

First challenge swim
Swim 10 lengths. Try to change stroke for 4th and 8th lengths only
Rest a maximum of 1 minute
Swim 5 lengths. Change stroke for 3rd length
Rest a maximum of 1 minute
Swim 5 lengths. Change stroke for 3rd length

Easy swim. Relax

For interest and future reference, try to check how long the full 20 lengths takes to swim. It is not essential to be too precise; an ordinary wall clock will suffice
If you complete this session fairly easily, try:

Second challenge swim
(After warm-up, as above)
Swim 10 lengths
Rest 1 minute
Repeat 10 lengths. Change stroke on 4th and 8th lengths
Again, if this is successful, try:

Third challenge swim
(After warm-up, as above)
Swim 20 lengths, continuous
Change stroke each 4th length for 1 length only
Again compare time of total swim

Session 7 **Warm-up**
4 lengths – 1st choice stroke
Rest 1 minute
4 × 1 length – alternate 2nd and 3rd choice strokes. These should be steady swims

Main training section. This is really the first of the interval-type sessions. Aim to perform each swim at the same speed and rhythm. Keeping the rest period between down to that indicated. The important thing is to start off at the right speed. This should be very controlled, with emphasis on a positive and full breathing pattern. If necessary, increase the rest towards the end of the set, but on subsequent sessions try to cut it down
2 lengths – 1st choice stroke
1 length – 2nd choice stroke
2 lengths – 1st choice stroke
1 length – 3rd choice stroke
2 lengths – 1st choice stroke
4 lengths – mixed strokes, and concentrate on good steady stroke technique

Easy swim

94

Session 8	**Warm-up.** As for Session 7

Main training section
2 × 2 lengths – 1st choice stroke
Rest 15–30 secs between each 2 lengths
1 length – 2nd choice stroke
Rest to recovery
4 lengths – 1st choice stroke
Rest to recovery
1 length – 3rd choice stroke
Rest to recovery
2 × 2 lengths – 1st choice stroke
Rest 15–30 secs between each 2 lengths

Easy swim. Relax and practise turns

Repeat this session once. Try to hold repeat swims at same speed, keeping to the same rest periods, and maintaining the style of stroke, trying not to allow it to become ragged

Session 9	**Warm-up.** As for Session 7

Main training section
3 × 2 lengths – 1st choice stroke
Rest 15–30 secs between each 2 lengths
1 length – 2nd choice stroke
Rest maximum 1 minute
4 lengths – 1st choice stroke
Rest maximum 1 minute
1 length – 3rd choice stroke
Rest maximum 1 minute
3 × 2 lengths – 1st choice stroke
Rest 15–30 secs between each 2 lengths

Easy swim. Relax

Try to hold repeat swims at same speed, with same rest and same stroke

Session 10	**Warm-up.** As for Section 7

Main training section
Aim to hold stroke and speed constant
4 lengths – 1st choice stroke
Rest 30–45 secs
3 lengths – 1st choice stroke
Rest 30 secs
2 lengths – 1st choice stroke
Rest 20 secs
1 length – 1st choice stroke
Rest to recovery
4 lengths – alternate 2nd and 3rd choice strokes
Rest to recovery

The following are stroke-development swims, so rest as required in order to swim correctly:
1 length – 1st choice stroke
1 length – 2nd choice stroke

1 length – 3rd choice stroke
1 length – 1st choice stroke

Easy swim. Relax. Practise turns

Session 11   **Warm-up**
1 length – 1st choice stroke
2 lengths – 2nd choice stroke
1 length – 1st choice stroke
2 lengths – 3rd choice stroke

Main training section
5 × 2 lengths – 1st choice stroke
Rest 15–30 secs between each 2 lengths
4 lengths – alternate 2nd and 3rd choice strokes
Rest to recovery
6 × 1 length – 1st choice stroke
Rest 10–20 secs between each length
4 lengths – alternate 2nd and 3rd choice strokes
Rest to recovery
2 lengths – 1st choice stroke

Easy swim. Relax

Session 12   **Warm-up**
4 lengths – mixed strokes
4 × 1 length – 1st choice stroke

Main training section
4 lengths – 1st choice stroke
1 length – 2nd choice stroke
4 lengths – 1st choice stroke
1 length – 3rd choice stroke
4 lengths – 1st choice stroke
1 length – 2nd choice stroke
4 lengths – 1st choice stroke
1 length – 3rd choice stroke
4 lengths – 1st choice stroke
Aim for 15–30 secs rest between all swims. And relax on
the 1 length swims as much as possible to prepare for a
good, steady effort on the 4 lengths

Easy swim. Relax

Sessions 11 and 12 both total 800 metres and at this
stage you are ready for more challenge swims

CHALLENGE   **Warm-up.** As for challenge swim 1

First challenge swim
Swim for 5 minutes, to the nearest length
Check time on clock and rest 30 secs to 1 minute
Repeat 5 mins swim
Rest 30 secs to 1 minute
Repeat 5 mins swim

Easy swim

Check the number of lengths on each 5 minutes swim
and compare. Then add total together. This total can
now be compared with:

96

Second challenge swim
(After warm-up as above)
Swim 15 minutes, to the nearest length, and check time
on clock

Easy swim

THE SWIMMER. This final level is the competent per-
former who has not only sound stroke techniques, but some
previous experience of training. Among the group may be
a number of people who are swimmers when much
younger, but have not done any training recently. Thus the
programme presents a full range of sessions from intro-
ductory to fairly intensive. Assess your level of fitness, and
'plug in' at the appropriate point. **Note:** The best plan is to
start a slight slot or two below your actual level and climb
up. This will produce not only a sense of satisfaction, but
the necessary adaptation far more comfortably. Good
luck, and many years of splendid swimming!

Session 1   **Warm-up.** Do not start off at too hard a pace, particularly if you have been away from swimming for even a
fairly short time. Remember that the various orientation
and adjustment practices outlined in previous levels,
might prove useful if you find yourself tiring or becoming breathless too soon:
1 length – 1st choice stroke
1 length – 2nd choice stroke
1 length – 1st choice stroke
1 length – 3rd choice stroke
Rest as required between each length until ready for the
next

Main training section
Repeat warm-up swims, this time aiming to rest slightly
less

Easy swim. Relax, practise turns

Repeat this session a couple of times, even though you
feel it is rather easy. It is a sound foundation on which to
build

Session 2   **Warm-up**
2 lengths – 1st and 2nd choice strokes
Rest as required
2 lengths – 1st and 3rd choice strokes

Main training section
1 length – 1st choice stroke
1 length – 2nd choice stroke
2 lengths – 1st choice stroke
1 length – 3rd choice stroke

97

2 lengths − 1st choice stroke
1 length − 2nd choice stroke
Rest to recovery between swims, and check how long
that takes

Easy swim. Relax, practise turns

Repeat this session until you can manage the 2 length
swims with no difficulty in breathing and you are resting
only about 1 minute maximum between swims

Session 3
Warm-up
4 lengths   − 1st, 2nd, 3rd, 1st choice strokes
4 × 1 length − same stroke order. These are stroke-
                development swims
Rest as required, and aim to perform strokes as effectively as possible

Main training section
2 lengths − 2nd choice stroke
4 lengths − 1st choice stroke
2 lengths − 3rd choice stroke
Rest as required between swims

Easy swim. Relax, practise turns

Repeat until you are able to do 4 lengths without stopping and are fairly comfortable

Session 4
Warm-up. As for Session 3

Main training section
2 × 2 lengths − 1st choice stroke
1 length   − 2nd choice stroke
4 lengths   − 1st choice stroke
2 lengths   − 3rd choice stroke
2 lengths   − 1st choice stroke
Rest for around 1 minute between each swim, but rest to
recovery before 4 lengths swim

Easy swim

Try to sustain a steady pace on each swim, and repeat if
unable to continue with only 1 minute rest between
swims

Session 5
Warm-up. As for Session 3

Main training section
4 lengths − 1st choice stroke
Rest 1 minute maximum
2 lengths − 2nd and 3rd choice strokes
Rest 1 minute maximum
3 × 2 lengths − 1st choice stroke
Rest 45 secs between each 2 lengths
2 lengths − 2nd and 3rd choice strokes
Rest to recovery
4 × 1 length − 1st choice stroke
Rest as required
These last 4 lengths are stroke-development swims. Aim
for good strokes

98

Easy swim

Repeat until able to hold rhythm and rest

Session 6   **Warm-up.** As for Session 3

Main training section
6 lengths – 1st choice stroke
Rest to recovery
2 lengths – 2nd choice stroke
Rest 50–60 secs
4 lengths – 1st choice stroke
Rest to recovery
2 lengths – 2nd and 3rd choice strokes
Rest 50–60 secs
2 lengths – 1st choice stroke
Rest to discovery
2 lengths – 2nd and 3rd choice strokes
Rest 50–60 secs
2 × 1 length – 1st choice stroke
Rest as required
Last 2 lengths – stroke development

Easy swim

Repeat until able to hold same stroke and speed throughout. You are now ready for some challenge swims

CHALLENGE   **Warm-up**
1 length – 1st choice stroke
2 lengths – 2nd and 3rd choice strokes
1 length – 1st choice stroke
Rest as required

First challenge swim
Swim 10 lengths – change stroke for 4th and 8th lengths
                         only
Rest a maximum of 1 minute
Swim 5 lengths – change stroke on 3rd length
Rest a maximum of 1 minute
Swim 5 lengths – change stroke on 3rd length

Easy swim

For interest and future reference, try to check how long
it takes to complete the 20 lengths
Record and compare with:

Second challenge swim
Swim 10 lengths – change stroke for 4th and 8th lengths
                         only
Rest a maximum of 1 minute
Swim 10 lengths – change stroke on 4th and 8th lengths

Easy swim

Again record the total time and compare with:

Third challenge swim
Swim 20 lengths continuously – change stroke each 4th
length for 1 length only

Again compare the time taken, and record for subsequent comparison

These three challenge swims should be attempted in sessions fairly close to each other for best effect, say over a two-week period. However, do not move on from the first or second challenge swim until you have achieved it without undue discomfort. If it was too difficult, move back to Session 6 and try again later. When you have successfully done all the challenge swims, you are ready to move on to the next set of sessions

Session 7

Warm-up

4 lengths   – 1st choice stroke, steady swim
4 × 1 length – 1st, 2nd, 3rd, 1st choice strokes
Rest as required
2 lengths – 1st choice stroke, preparation for main section

Main training section
4 × 2 lengths – 1st choice stroke
Rest 30–45 secs between each 2 lengths
2 lengths – 2nd choice stroke
Rest to recovery
4 lengths – 1st choice stroke
Rest to recovery
2 lengths – 3rd choice stroke
Rest to recovery
4 × 1 length – 1st choice stroke
Rest 30 secs between each length

Easy swim

Aim to hold each of the 2 length repeats at the same speed with the same rest if possible. It is vital to start off at a controlled pace, with emphasis on regular and positive breathing

Repeat this session once

Session 8

Warm-up. As for Session 7

Main training section
2 × 4 lengths – 1st choice stroke
Rest 40–50 secs between each 4 lengths
2 × 2 lengths – 2nd and 3rd choice strokes
Rest 50–60 secs between each 2 lengths
4 × 2 lengths – 1st, 2nd, 1st, 3rd choice strokes
Rest 30–45 secs between each 2 lengths
4 × 1 length – 1st choice stroke, stroke development
Rest as required

Easy swim

Session 9

Warm-up. As for Session 7

Main training section
8 lengths – 1st choice stroke
Rest 30–60 secs
2 lengths – 2nd choice stroke
Rest to recovery

100

6 lengths – 1st choice stroke
Rest 30–60 secs
2 lengths – 3rd choice stroke
Rest to recovery
4 lengths – 1st choice stroke
Rest 30–60 secs
2 lengths – 2nd and 3rd choice strokes
Rest to recovery
2 lengths – 1st choice stroke
Rest to discovery
4 × 1 length – 2nd choice stroke, stroke development
Rest as required

Easy swim. Relax, practise turns

Session 10   **Warm-up.** As for Session 7

Main training section
1 length – 1st choice stroke
2 lengths – 1st choice stroke
3 lengths – 1st choice stroke
4 lengths – 2nd choice stroke
3 lengths – 1st choice stroke
2 lengths – 1st choice stroke
Rest – aim to keep rest to a maximum of 30 secs between swims
1 length – 1st choice stroke
Rest to recovery
4 × 1 length – 3rd choice stroke, stroke development
Rest as required
5 × 2 lengths – 1st choice stroke
Rest 15–30 secs between each 2 lengths

Easy swim

Try to hold a steady pace on each swim. Repeat until able to hold pace and rest as well as stroke throughout

Session 11   **Warm-up.** As for Session 7

Main training section
3 × 4 lengths – 1st choice stroke
Rest 30–60 secs between each 4 lengths
4 lengths – alternate 2nd and 3rd choice stroke
Rest to recovery
8 lengths – 1st choice stroke
Rest to recovery
5 × 2 lengths – 1st, 2nd, 1st, 3rd, 1st choice strokes
Rest 15–45 secs between each 2 lengths

Easy swim

Repeat until able to hold speed to your satisfaction, maintain stroke pattern and rest within maximum limits set

Session 12   **Warm-up.** As for Session 7

Main training section
3 × 10 lengths – 4 lengths 1st choice stroke

101

1 length 2nd choice stroke
1 length 3rd choice stroke
4 lengths 1st choice stroke
Rest for 1 minute between each set
4 × 2 lengths – 1st choice stroke, 2nd choice stroke
1st choice stroke, 3rd choice stroke
These are stroke development swims, so rest as required

Easy swim

When you can manage this session without difficulty, you are ready for more challenge swims

CHALLENGE **Warm-up**
8 lengths – steady swim, change strokes
Rest as required
2 × 1 length – stroke check
Rest as required

First challenge swim
Swim 20 lengths continuous, every 5th length a different stroke
Rest 1 minute
Swim 15 lengths continuous, every 5th length a different stroke
Rest 1 minute
Swim 15 lengths continuous, changing strokes at will

For interest and future reference, check time of each section and also the overall time for 50 lengths

Easy swim

Second challenge swim
Swim 25 lengths, continuous, every 5th length a different stroke
Rest 1 minute
Swim 25 lengths continuous, changing strokes at will
Again check and record, and compare time taken overall

Easy swim

Third challenge swim
Swim 50 lengths continuously, changing strokes at will

Check, record and compare overall times

These challenge swims should be attempted over a two-week period. However, do not move on from first or second challenge swim until you can manage without excessive difficulty. Should this be so, move back to Session 12 and try again later. When you have successfully done all the challenge swims, you are ready to move to the next set of sessions. These are suitable for people in training to participate in competitions, such as Masters (veterans) tournaments

Session 13 **Warm-up**
2 lengths   – 1st choice stroke
4 × 1 length – 1st, 2nd, 1st, 3rd choice stroke

102

Rest as required
4 lengths – 1st, 2nd, 3rd, 1st choice stroke
These swims are to be used to adjust to the water, so swim very steadily and emphasise breathing

Main training section
3 × 4 lengths – 1st choice stroke, holding stroke and
                    speed steady
Rest 30–60 secs between each 4 lengths
4 lengths – 2nd and 3rd choice strokes
Rest as required
4 × 2 lengths – 1st choice stroke
Rest 20–30 secs between each 2 lengths
4 lengths – 2nd and 3rd choice strokes
Rest as required
4 × 1 length – 1st choice stroke
Try to swim each of these singles slightly faster, resting as required between each length

Easy swim. Practise turns

Session 14   **Warm-up.** As for Session 13

Main training section
2 × 6 lengths – 2 lengths – 1st choice stroke
                      2 lengths – 2nd choice stroke
                      2 lengths – 1st choice stroke
Rest 30–60 secs, then:
2 lengths – 1st choice stroke
2 lengths – 3rd choice stroke
2 lengths – 1st choice stroke
6 lengths – alternate 2nd and 3rd choice strokes
Rest as required
2 × 4 lengths – 1st choice stroke
Rest 20–45 secs between each 4 lengths
2 × 4 lengths – 1st, 2nd, 3rd, 1st choice strokes
Try to swim slightly faster on 2nd length of each swim, and rest as required

Easy swim

Session 15   **Warm-up.** As for Session 13

Main training section
10 lengths – 2 lengths – 1st choice stroke
                2 lengths – 2nd choice stroke
                2 lengths – 1st choice stroke
                2 lengths – 3rd choice stroke
                2 lengths – 1st choice stroke
Swim steadily on 2nd and 3rd choice strokes, but try to swim faster on 1st choice stroke
4 × 2 lengths – 1st choice stroke
Hold pace and stroke on each swim and rest for 15–30 secs between each 2 lengths
6 lengths – alternate 2nd and 3rd choice strokes, steady swim
6 × 1 length 1st choice stroke, stroke development

103

Rest 10–20 secs between each length, but if required take an additional 30 secs after 3 lengths, and then return to 10–20 secs rest
4 lengths – 2nd, 3rd, 2nd, 3rd choice strokes, steady swim

Easy swim

Session 16

Warm-up
1 length – 3rd choice stroke
2 lengths – 2nd choice stroke
3 lengths – 1st choice stroke
2 lengths – 2nd choice stroke
1 length – 3rd choice stroke
1 length – 1st choice stroke, stroke development
Rest as required between first three swims, and try to cut down rest on the others

Main training section
5 × 2 lengths – 1st choice stroke
Rest 15–30 secs between each 2 lengths
4 lengths – 2nd choice stroke
Rest to recovery
3 × 4 lengths – each 4 length swim consists of:
        1 length – 1st choice stroke
        1 length – 2nd choice stroke
        1 length – 3rd choice stroke
        1 length – 1st choice stroke
Rest 30–60 secs between each 4 lengths
4 lengths – 3rd choice stroke
Rest to recovery
10 × 1 length – alternate 1st and 2nd choice strokes
Rest 30–60 secs between each length

Easy swim

Session 17

Warm-up. As for Session 16

Main training section
8 lengths – alternate 2 lengths 2nd and 3rd choice strokes
Rest to recovery
2 × 4 lengths – 1st choice stroke
Rest 30–60 secs between each 4 lengths
8 lengths – alternate lengths, 2nd and 3rd choice strokes
Rest to recovery
4 × 2 lengths – 1st choice stroke
Rest 15–30 secs between each 2 lengths
8 × 1 length – alternate lengths, 2nd, 1st, 2nd, 3rd choice stroke, etcetera, i.e. use your 2nd choice stroke on odd-number lengths, and alternate your 1st and 3rd choice strokes on the even-number lengths
Rest 60 secs between each length

Easy swim

Session 18

Warm-up. As for Session 16

Main training section
10 lengths – 1st choice stroke

104

Rest to recovery
5 × 2 lengths – 2nd choice stroke
Rest 30–60 secs between each 2 lengths
10 lengths – 3rd choice stroke
Rest to recovery
5 × 2 lengths – 1st choice stroke
Rest 15–30 secs between each 2 lengths
10 lengths – 2nd choice stroke

Easy swim

Repeat this session until able to do all swims with ease, and resting as indicated or even less
You are now ready for more challenge swims

CHALLENGE **Warm-up**
4 lengths – any stroke
4 × 1 length – 1st choice stroke
Rest as required

First challenge swim
Swim 32 lengths (800 metres)
Check and record time taken to complete
Rest 1–2 minutes, or as required
Swim 28 lengths (700 metres)
Check and record time taken to complete

Easy swim

Combine the two times to give an overall 1,500-metre time, and on the basis of this time set yourself a target for:

Second challenge swim
Swim 1,500 metres, continuous
Check time, compare with target and record for future comparison

CHAPTER TEN

In the Pool

The extraordinary thing about Britain is that, despite the fact that we have so many swimming pools, their use for fitness is so little realised. People who wish actually to exercise in a pool find that it is often almost impossible to do so because it is being used for recreational romping about rather than swimming. There is a constant danger of being jumped on, and little chance of being able to make an unimpeded course down the pool.

There is a great deal of good in this joyful use of water, and pools catering for this are now being built in free-form shapes. What is wrong is that so little attention is paid to the requirements of exercise swimmers who are not competitive club members. Looking after *them*, will help improve the general health of the community.

Contrast the British attitude to that of the Dutch. There a national four-day swimming event is now held every year. The idea started in the town of Deventer in 1970, with the object of encouraging people to swim a specific distance each day. Within five years, the four-day event had become a national occasion, and now over a quarter of a million people take part. The participants attempt to swim 500 metres on each of the four days, and each swimmer who completes 2,000 metres is given a medal.

During the event, local swimming baths become focal points for local people, providing an opportunity for other activities as well as swimming. There are exhibitions, demonstrations, fashion shows and discos. Crucially, the event is *not* a competition: there is no emphasis on the time taken to swim the distance, only on completing it. What it helps to instil is the idea of *regular swimming for health reasons*.

It is strange that in Britain we take such care to see that

children are taught to swim but fail to follow through into adult life. The most voluble adult voices are all too often those that complain about the cost of running swimming pools. Irate ratepayers complain that they do not make money, as if swimming pools, unlike parks and public libraries, should be commercial concerns showing a nice profit at the end of the year.

What really should be questioned is not financial profit, but whether pools are being properly programmed so that full use is made of them. A place where the word 'programming' is heard frequently is at Copthall, in North London, where Barnet Borough Council has built a complex for swimmers that is probably the finest in Europe: two pools each 25 metres in length and in which a normal-sized adult can stand at any point, plus a pool for diving and synchronised swimming.

The inspiration for the Copthall complex is largely to the credit of Barnet's baths manager, Alan Hime, a former leading swimming coach and a man with vision that knows no bounds when it comes to helping people to swim. He believes the crucial consideration with any pool is how you allocate time within it. Too many pools allow use by all and sundry most of the time. As a result, many people are put off early in a pool's life. All too frequently, their experience is an unfortunate one: the pool is crowded with kids or adults or both, with everybody swimming here, there and everywhere, plus diving and jumping. And in the end, what can happen is that the pool can become grossly under-used, often empty, at a time when a specified group could be making full use of it.

It is hard to imagine such unrestricted use being allowed within any other sporting facility. Think of the chaos that would ensue on a running track if some people ran round the wrong way! What is the answer? The psychology of the situation reminds me of the great Wilkinson razor-blade boom. The blade became popular when it was in short supply, which some said was a calculated tactic of the manufacturers. Whatever the truth, there is no question that many men considered it a favour to be able to buy these blades from their hairdresser. The same tactic can be equally well applied to a pool: allocate times so that people feel privileged when they are using it, whether they are women enjoying a housewives' social swim, children a family session, mothers a babies' class, or senior citizens a period for themselves.

Experience shows that programming of these proportions encourages rather than deters adults and children to turn up at specific periods, knowing that they will be able to enjoy the pool in a way they can look forward to. But it is still the exception rather than the rule. Copthall is a pacesetter, both because of Alan Hime and because, as a new establishment, it can more easily introduce innovations. The best idea of the lot may be the two lanes Copthall has permanently reserved in one pool for exercise swimmers.

Except at places like Copthall, the *pleasure* of physical activity is still very rarely well promoted in Britain today. Somehow the cold-shower concept has invaded our national consciousness so thoroughly that an extra effort is now needed to persuade people that exercise is actually pleasant. And the voices that speak out in this area need to be better publicised.

Doc Counsilman, the American swimming coach mentioned earlier in this book, is in his fifties, but he still swims regularly and well. He does not obscure his personal joy in the swimming jargon of a coach. To him, it is simple. Like many other members of his generation, and of a younger generation, he used to imagine himself swimming a powerful crawl stroke like Johnny Weismuller did in Tarzan films. 'When I finally did learn to swim the crawl stroke efficiently, and was swimming it in a high-school meet,' Counsilman said, 'the feeling I got was just as I had imagined it would be. Even today, as a coach, I swim about two miles a day, most of it crawl stroke. I still get that enjoyable feeling of rhythm and power as I go through the water . . . Many people get this feeling when they swim.'

Preparing for the water

If you are ready to get into the pool and swim for fitness

and pleasure, there are a few warnings to note first. Clearly, people with coronary heart disease should not go leaping into cold water. Anyone who is prone to attacks of intermittent unconsciousness – such as an epileptic – should not go swimming, even in warm water, unless accompanied by a competent swimmer. And people with ear problems such as perforated eardrums should not go swimming at all.

Before the training schedules, I said that if you are over 35 and unsure of your fitness, or have had a major illness, you should first of all check with your doctor before taking up reasonably strenuous exercise. You *cannot* be too careful, but an argument has been propounded by various authorities recently which underlines that most of us are our own best guide. This is not simply because so many ordinary general practitioners are not experienced in assessing people's capability for physical exercise (or that GPs nationwide might be inundated with requests for exercise clearance) but because it is now felt that, provided you *feel* well, and do not start a programme of exercise at a level that is beyond you, there is a greater risk in non-activity. The Health Education Council propounded in a recent campaign:

In general, the long-term health hazards of not exercising are more serious than the short-term risks associated with fitness schemes. With proper safety precautions, no serious harm should come to anyone.

1. If you are under 35, start training as soon as possible, but take it gradually at first.

2. If you are over 35 and under 50, and you have not taken exercise since you left school, you can start to exercise gradually, but if you are worried about exercise symptoms, consult your doctor.

3. If you are over 50, you should seek medical advice before starting a fitness scheme. You cannot harm yourself by walking too much, and you may be able to start more energetic activities.

The emphasis, as you see, is on starting at an exercise

level which you can handle. *Do not* be egged on by unthinking enthusiasts, who should know better, to do something which makes you feel uncomfortable on the basis of their advice that it will 'do you good'. The chances are that it will not. Commence at a stage which is beyond you, and you may well give up because you will not be enjoying yourself. You can even do yourself a great deal of harm. It is better to start at a lower level and benefit from the resulting boost you will receive from your quick progress.

Never expect to 'get in shape' overnight, because physical conditioning should occur in a well-graduated way. The body takes time to get used to the demands of exercise. For this very reason, always take account, when assessing yourself, of such variables as the weather, fatigue, recent illness and stress. If you are forced, possibly by illness to lay-off, never attempt to perform at pre-lay-off levels; you will have plenty in hand, so you will come back quickly enough.

Remember again that the spacing out of exercise is important. American writer Hal Higdon in a book he wrote called *Fitness After Forty*, quotes Dr. Noel D. Nequin, director of a cardiac rehabilitation centre. Nequin's advice is borne out by much experience: 'In order to maintain your fitness level, you must reinforce your body with exercise every 60 hours. We used to say a minimum of three days a week was necessary. Now we talk more about four days a week, because that comes closer to the ideal of never resting more than 60 hours (2½ days) between exercise.'

Since most women's hearts and lung capacities are smaller, a woman may do less than a man each time she exercises, but spacing out the sessions is equally important.

When exercising, the pulse rate, of course, rather than your state of breathlessness, is the guide. The average person needs to sustain a heart beat of 150 to the minute for the exercise to produce the necessary training effect within the time allowed. If the pulse rate is less, then you have to extend the exercise.

However, to check that you are working up to your goal in a graduated fashion, take your pulse five minutes after

110

exercise. If it's still over 120 a minute, it is a sign that the exercise was too tough. Ten minutes after exercise, your pulse should be back below 100. If it is not, you should let up a little on your exercise programme. An average resting pulse rate is about 70. As you exercise, your base rate, best taken in the morning when you wake up, will drop, perhaps to 50 or below. Don't worry if it does not fall as low as other people's. Some people have naturally slower heart rates.

You can measure your pulse rate (though don't become obsessive about it) in a pool most easily by placing the index or middle finger on the carotid artery on the neck and under the jaw, or simply by placing the hand on the chest under the breast and slightly to the left. If you have been working-out, you will have no trouble in feeling the beat. Take it as soon as you stop, because once you rest, the heartbeat immediately starts to drop. Look at a clock, take the beat for 10 seconds and by multiplying by six you will have your pulse rate.

In starting regular swimming, you are in for a pleasant surprise if you have never trained regularly before because you are almost bound to improve beyond any performance you may have put up when you were younger. Whatever your age and experience, remember you will find in the pool that you can always continue to learn and improve your skill and technique.

Gerald Forsberg, the former English Channel swimmer whom we tested at St. Mary's College, has for instance a best mile time of 26 minutes 40 seconds. He swam this in 1952. He could still swim, at 65, a mile in 31 minutes 40 seconds, or equivalent to a less than the approximate one per cent deterioration in performance per year measured among many veteran swimmers after their peak. 'That time is 84 per cent of my former speed,' said Forsberg. 'However, it is not what I might be doing, partly because I am not doing the training today and secondly, I've got two stone more weight on me than before. It's like having a bigger ship to drive through the water with the same engine. Weight is not a function of age really. I could take off the

111

two stone and obviously my speed would be better. On the whole, I think you could say that a 65-year-old could be 90 per cent as good as at his peak.'

So take advantage of any coaching when you can and, if you feel the need, join a club. And remember the water is a world of infinite possibilities.

What to wear

There is no question that swimwear is more of a problem for women than men. If you are a man, the advice I can give is simple. You may feel that 'racing' briefs made of light nylon are for competitive swimmers only, and it would embarrass you to wear them. Certainly, I would not persuade anyone to wear something they feel uncomfortable in. If you are, to begin with, a bit fat, you may even feel happiest of all in a pair of the boxer-type shorts that are made as much for the beach as for the water. However, as you grow more confident and attain the shape you are aiming at, you will almost certainly find nylon briefs the most satisfactory wear for the water. Too many other swimming trunks are made of material that is heavy when wet and does not dry out very quickly.

There is a feeling of freedom and lack of weight that nylon briefs provide, as well as two other important points to consider. Firstly, if you are swimming frequently, it is convenient to have swimwear that *will* dry rapidly. Secondly, such lightweight swimwear can be folded, put into a small plastic bag and slipped easily into a hip pocket. This means that if you are willing to hire a towel at a pool, you can be constantly equipped for a swim, unencumbered by a large bag.

The explosion, incidentally, in the 'leisure' market has awakened firms who specialise in 'competition' wear like Speedo, Arena and Bukta, to a new potential. They are now making less-sparsely-cut men's briefs and women's suits that take account of fuller figures, in the same lightweight materials they have always used. But finding suitable swimwear for a middle-aged overweight or large-bosomed lady is still not easy, which is a pity since so many women find swimming an ideal way to get fit.

How many more women would be in the pool if only they could find suitable swimsuits? The problem is a perfectly natural and understandable one. Women who are out of shape do not want to make this obvious. They would rather 'look their best' but balancing these considerations against the available choice presents a conundrum, because the two influences in the manufacturing area, competition and fashion requirements, are in conflict.

Now that the two influences have come together somewhat in the 'leisure' ranges of the competition swimwear manufacturers, women taking up swimming seriously for exercise would be well advised to try on before buying. If you still find that these suits make you feel uncomfortable because they stretch across the body too much, and make you look like a tadpole, then a more 'fashionable' suit found in a fashion or department store is bound to be more comfortable because it is going to provide more support.

But remember that you are looking all the time for something that is going to be athletically functional. Therefore, reject halterneck straps, which are impractical for vigorous swimming, and ensure that the suit does not 'gap' too much at the top, or it will catch the water. It is likely that the ideal all-round-suit will be made from nylon for basic strength. When you try on a suit, check that the straps, and where the garment fits round the legs, stay comfortable when you move.

Both women and men should always remember that swimwear lasts longer for being rinsed out in fresh water after use. It is not chlorine that causes the rot to set in, incidentally, but sweat. Working hard in a pool you will sweat, though you may not be aware of it.

Swimming caps these days are uni-sex items, apart from the flower-petal creations one sometimes sees. If you need to keep the hair dry and out of your face, Speedo swimhats come in several shades of latex. Speedo also make two-colour Lycra hats. All in one size, they stretch to fit any

113

head. Nevertheless, women may need to experiment, particularly if they have long hair.

If you suffer from *otitis externa*, a mild but painful inflammation of the outer ear, caused by water carrying infection into it, you will need ear plugs. Britain's Olympic gold medallist, David Wilkie, has suffered recurring bouts of otitis himself. He recommends the wax-ball type of plug because it can be pressed into a shape for you alone, and then retained for several uses.

● **Goggles.** Wilkie won his Olympic medals wearing goggles, and helped make them so popular. Now thousands upon thousands of froggy-eyed swimmers plough up and down British pools. There is, however, a case that needs to be stated against wearing goggles. No evidence has been produced that chlorinated water can damage the eye. Soreness from swimming is caused by water of any sort washing away the natural fluids that bathe our eyes. This can affect the sight badly enough to blur the accuracy needed in driving or playing a ball game, but only temporarily. And though chlorine may irritate the eye, conjunctivitis is usually passed on by shared towels in the changing room.

On the other hand, severe eye injuries can be caused by goggles. The typical accident reported in medical journals results from incorrect handling. When children pull goggles straight out from the face to clean them, the goggles can snap back so violently on the strong elastic straps that they lacerate the eyeball. The Royal Society for the Prevention of Accidents has published a poster showing the safe way to remove goggles: sliding them up on to the forehead, then taking them off the top of the head. *Always* use both hands to avoid danger of twisting the eyepieces.

Diving into the water in goggles is not recommended. This is because, to fit well, they must be snug around the eyeball, and touching all the soft parts around the eye; extra pressure caused by diving could hurt and seriously bruise. There is, in addition, a certain amount of draw on the eyeball.

Let me now say that many people, myself included, have found goggles a godsend. Before I wore them, to swim for any extended period in a pool left my eyes sore. After a session in an over-chlorinated bath, I was invariably left with eyes that felt as if a needle was sticking into each pupil. It was difficult actually to keep the eyes open in such circumstances. They would water so much that people commented on the fact. Goggles have put an end to this misery.

So if you need goggles, what should one look for? The *Sunday Times* organised a test in which several swimmers took part, testing over a period of time almost every type of goggle on the market. The survey paid particular attention to comfort; how much water they let in, if any; range of vision; and how badly, initially and consistently, they misted up.

Comfort depends largely on the shape of your head, so you should try on the goggles in the shop. Well-padded rims tend to be more comfortable, but how much water goggles let in was shown in the test to depend on the snugness of the fit. Models made entirely of non-cellular plastic were not only less efficient – they were uncomfortable and sometimes painful. The cellular padding on other models was better when it was sturdy as opposed to squashy.

What people forget, particularly when trying on goggles in a shop, is to take advantage of the adjustments that can be made to straps, and especially to the bridge-piece across the nose. But remember always to make adjustments away from the water and with dry hands so that there is no danger of the goggles snapping back and possibly damaging your eyes. Though tiresome sometimes to fiddle with bridge-pieces, especially where young, excited children are involved, it is essential to get the adjustments right.

The range of vision in goggles is generally good regardless of shape. Being able to see clearly in the water, apart from the protection afforded the eye, is another good reason for wearing them. In a busy pool, goggles make it less likely that you will bump into somebody. Untinted goggles are easier to see through at all times, tinted lenses being of value only in sunnier climates than Britain's. But if you like the look of tinted goggles, the amount of effect they have on vision is not enough to be troublesome.

The worst problem with all goggles is that they mist up. Most people counter this by spitting – not in disgust, but to coat each eyepiece with saliva. If you allow them to mist up once, then lick the inside of the goggles, the second misting is less severe. You can also try the trick of soaking a pair in neat liquid detergent overnight, then rinsing. It does make a great improvement.

Much the best I have come across are called Aqua-See, which are imported from America by Norville Optical Ltd., of Gloucester. Unfortunately, they can be obtained only through an optician. The Aqua-See have take-out lenses that can be ground to a prescription if you normally wear spectacles, but they are also supplied with plain lenses. Not surprisingly they are comparatively expensive, at least seven times the cost of the best British goggles, called Sportsgear, which come with a double strap to hold them more efficiently in place.

But whatever goggles you buy, particularly if you decide on a cheaper model, check that the word 'shatterproof' or 'unbreakable' is on the pack. (Sportsgear goggles, for example, will withstand a bashing from a hammer.) And remember to always feel for sharp edges on frames.

● **Kickboards.** There are other swimming aids on the market, including hand paddles which help to strengthen the arms and develop a correct arm stroke, but the only other item you will need if you are going to follow the training schedules in this book fully is a kickboard. The best are marketed by World of Service UK and are made in water-resistant high and low density polyethylene which makes them sufficiently rigid, yet resilient. They are made in Junior, Senior and Olympic sizes, but for most normal-sized adults, the Senior kickboard, which is 21 inches long, $10\frac{1}{2}$ inches wide and 1 inch thick is quite big enough for using on leg-kick practice. This board is too big, though, for gripping between the thighs on arms-only drills, and you will need the smaller Junior kickboard for this, or a Speedo polystyrene swim float, which is cheaper. Alternatively, World of Service UK market a Pull-Buoy, consisting of two cylinders of polyethylene which are attached just above the knees. Details of this equipment and other items are best obtained direct from World of Service UK, since it is basically a mail order outfit. They will send their current prices if you write to them at PO Box No. 48, Harpenden, Herts. AL5 3AX.

CHAPTER ELEVEN

Out of the Pool

More theories have been expounded about the diets of swimmers than most other subjects under the sun. But if you are not aiming for an Olympic medal, you can get by without expert advice. The dictum is clear: eat sensibly.

If you regularly spread your bread liberally with butter, take sugar in your tea and coffee, eat quantities of cream cakes and daily consume breakfasts of bacon, eggs and sausages, the adjustment will be drastic. If this is not the case, then the chances are your diet will not need to change a great deal. Any excess in your intake may simply be 'burned off' in exercise.

The most important thing is that your diet should be well-balanced. 'A little of what you fancy does you good' may be what grandmother said, but it is as true today as it ever was. The emphasis should be placed on the word little, because we live in a society where people tend to grow up over-eating. A baby at the breast knows when it has had enough; a built-in signalling system ensures this. But as soon as that baby is old enough to comprehend language, a doting mother can convince a child that 'eating up' and consequently over-eating, is tantamount to being good.

It is a vicious circle. The mother's love is confirmed for her by seeing her child eat. The child is equally convinced it is doing right by eating up, since it clearly makes the mother happy. The consequences in later life are disastrous: in Britain, up to one-third of the population is overweight, and too many children and adolescents are too fat.

If anything helps in breaking the over-eating habit, it is exercise. Physical activity not only burns up calories, but also, in time, dulls the desire to eat large quantities. The stomach gets smaller, the waist pulls in, and rather than leave the table feeling swollen you get up knowing you could have eaten more. You enjoy your food more, and in greater variety, but you eat less. In achieving this, exercise beats all the slimming systems hands down.

One of the reasons is that slimming programmes often advocate eating certain foods while ignoring others. This can be dangerous because it is important to eat different types of food; our bodies need a variety of vitamins if they are to function efficiently.

I wrote in an earlier chapter about the courses introduced at the Bath Sports Centre by the district community physician. A dietary talk I attended there for a group of middle-aged men was given by a charming Chinese lady. She distributed a simple guide to eating for health, prepared by a state registered dietician of Bath Health District and it contains as good advice as any I have ever seen. I am grateful to have been permitted to reproduce it here:

MEAT

Choose lean meat, and cut off all the fat that you can. Eat more poultry (e.g. chicken). Eat less pork, bacon, ham, beef, lamb. One meat meal a day is a good rule.

Grill meat rather than fry it. Roast chickens and joints in foil without adding fat. Pour away fat before making gravy.

FISH

All kinds of fish can be eaten. Try fresh, smoked, frozen and tinned fishes. Eat fish in place of meat for main meals.

Fry fish in corn oil or sunflower seed oil. Grill it with a little soft margarine. Bake it with skimmed milk or tomato juice. Serve poached fish with margarine instead of butter.

CHEESE

Cottage cheese can be used for salads and for stuffing tomatoes. Edam cheese has a lower fat content than Cheddar or Stilton. Try to restrict the higher-fat cheeses to two ounces a week.

Flavour cottage cheese with salt and pepper, chopped onions, chive, pineapple or celery to give variety.

EGGS

Eat no more than three whole eggs a week. These can be used in cakes or puddings, or taken as the basis of a main meal.

Egg-white and meringue is not restricted.

MILK

Fresh milk can be used for tea and coffee. Avoid using the top of the milk and cream.

Skimmed milk or dried milk (e.g. Marvel) can be used for making soups, sauces, custards and puddings.

VEGETABLES

Eat as much as you like of fresh and frozen vegetables. These are better food value than tinned vegetables.

Peas and beans and lentils can help to add protein to the diet.

SALADS

All salad vegetables can be eaten. Try cabbage, endive, chicory or Chinese leaves in place of lettuce.

Use oil and vinegar or lemon juice as a dressing. Try low-fat yoghurt as a dressing.

FRUIT

Eat as much fresh fruit as you can afford. Eat the skins of apples, pears, plums, etc. Avoid tinned fruit in syrup.

Fresh or stewed fruit makes a delicious start to breakfast. Try prunes, dried fruit salad and dried apricots.

STARCHES AND SUGARS

Choose wholemeal bread or crispbreads in place of white or brown bread. Eat plain rather than sweet biscuits. Choose porridge, muesli or wholewheat breakfast cereals (e.g. Weetabix, All Bran, Bran Buds, Shredded Wheat). Use sugar in cooking, but avoid putting it into drinks.

Try using wholewheat flour for making cakes, pastry, crumble toppings, etc. Delicious muesli can be made at home with porridge oats, dried fruit, grated apple and low-fat yoghurt.

FATS

Use corn oil or sunflower seed oil for cooking. Use Flora, St. Michael Supersoft, J.S. Special, Blueband or Kraft Soft Margarine in place of butter or lard.

Cooking oils labelled 'Vegetable Oil' are NOT suitable. Avoid lard, dripping, butter, cream and hard margarines.

DRINKS

Try to take at least eight cups of water a day. Avoid 'cokes', lemonade and sweetened fruit squashes.

Take fluid as tea, coffee, soup or fruit juice if you do not like water. Artificial tablets or liquid sweeteners can be used in place of sugar.

The emphasis in any sensible diet designed to help you to become fitter and healthier, the dietician in Bath told her audience, is firstly on the need to cut down on animal fats. These are present not only in meat, but in eggs, cream, cheese and butter. You can also help yourself achieve this by switching to poly-unsaturated fats, which, like the margarines suggested in the foregoing guide, are semi-solid or liquid at normal room temperature; solid margarines contain saturated fats, found in animal fats, so are not a substitute.

Secondly, there is a need to reduce the consumption of refined sugar, which in Britain is tremendous. In Britain, it is estimated each person spends, on average, around £1 a week on sweets and cakes for themselves or their family. The effect of sugar is to give you energy but no nourishment. You therefore burn up the sugar instead of other food you have eaten, and get fat. Finally, there is a distinct need to introduce roughage into the diet, everything from apples and cabbage to bran.

If you do want to slim, and bearing in mind what I have said about the body's reliance on a variety of foods, you simply eat smaller quantities of meat, fish, eggs, milk and cheese, and increase the amount of vegetables and salads. You cut down on bread, potatoes and fats, and leave out such high-calorie foods as sugar and sweets.

In considering your overall diet the point is quite straightforward, whether you are attempting to lose weight or not: The closer your food is to its natural state, the better. The more food is refined, the less likelihood there is that it will do you any good. The simplest example is the contrast between a good wholemeal loaf, and the white, pappy bread that does not deserve even the name. Wholemeal stimulates your saliva secretion because it needs to be chewed; it is therefore properly digested. White and pappy bread can't effectively be chewed; you swallow it in small lumps and it makes you constipated and put on weight. Your teeth, too, get less of a work-out with refined foods and thus they are also bad for them and your gums.

So far, I have not mentioned alcohol. In Bath only one small drink a day was suggested, 'if liked'. Certainly, alcohol has a high calorific content and should be avoided as much as possible if you are trying to lose weight. But I am not so sure that it is necessary to good health and fitness to be quite so abstemious – if you like to drink a little more. In fact, some recent evidence indicates that alcohol may do you some positive good *in moderation*. The United States Institute of Health has suggested that men who drink 12 glasses of wine a week, or the equivalent in beer and spirits, have a lower risk of coronary thrombosis than total abstainers. And Survival Kit, a subscription-only newsletter started by a fitness enthusiast in London, concluded after a review of the available evidence: 'Alcohol in moderation is relaxing, bactericidal, good for the digestion, a tonic for the circulation and an aid to longevity.'

At St. Mary's College, in Twickenham, after our swimmers had finished their tests and sat down to a meal together, most of them drank some wine. The rules can always occasionally be broken.

The cloud over smoking

If some satisfaction can be gained from the immediately previous conclusion by the moderate drinker, I am afraid there is nothing that can be said to console the smoker. There is only one thing basically to be said about smoking and that is *DON'T*.

My own aversion to smoking is lifelong. It was underlined by what cigarettes did to my father, who took up smoking long before the dangerous consequences were known. He died as a result of cigarette smoking, having for some time been barely able to walk a yard without stopping to catch his breath.

It is a killing business. Smoking damages the cardiovascular, respiratory and digestive systems, and encourages the growth of cancer in many parts of the body. Premature death is the prospect for anyone who risks the cigarette: Smokers are twice as likely to die before middle-age as non-smokers, and two out of five smokers die before 65, compared with only one of five non-smokers.

The chairman of the Tobacco Advisory Committee said in 1977: 'We must teach people to smoke sensibly.' This is impossible. The habit is addictive, which has been proved by injecting neat nicotine into smokers suffering withdrawal symptoms associated with giving up nicotine. After injection, the symptoms were quelled.

Swimming can alleviate the effects of smoking, and may even help a person to give up the habit. But lungs loaded with the effects of tobacco do not work well for their owners if they take up strenuous exercise. Remember that. And remember also, if you are in your mid-thirties and a smoker, your life expectancy is five and a half years shorter than a non-smoker's.

Do you really think anybody can smoke sensibly?

Facing up to life

Finally, let me emphasise that fitness, whether derived from swimming or any other strenuous exercise, helps you to know yourself, not only in a physical sense but a philosophical one also.

Physically, you become attuned to signals your body transmits to the brain much more clearly. You know, with much more accuracy, when to rest and when to press. It is easy to understand why this should be so: small electrical impulses pass continually between our contracting muscles, our moving joints and our brains when we exercise.

But understanding how fitness helps us to face up to ourselves is more difficult. One inspirationalist has explained it by saying that the athletic person has 'developed a sense of time, an acceptance of pain, an appreciation of relationships and a happiness that . . . completes him.' And if this is true for a runner, how much more this must mean for the swimmer in the water. It is where life began and if one day I find I cannot run, I never expect not to be able to swim. The water will support me.

References

Enjoying Rude Health, Robin Clarke, *Telegraph Magazine*, July 1975.

Aerobics, Kenneth H. Cooper, Bantam edition, 1968.

The New Aerobics, Kenneth H. Cooper, Bantam edition, 1970.

Aerobics For Women, Mildred Cooper and Kenneth H. Cooper, Bantam edition, 1973.

Doc Counsilman on Swimming, James E. Counsilman, Pelham, 1978.

Women: tadpole or siren?, Norman Harris, *The Sunday Times*, June 1976.

Fitness After Forty, Hal Higdon, World Publications (USA), 1977.

Benefits of Swimming to Heart and Lungs (and other articles), Paul Hutinger, *Master Swimmers Lane 4* (USA), 1977.

Running and Swimming World Records, P. Jokl and E. Jokl, *British Journal of Sports Medicine*, 1976.

The Medical Risks of Life, Stephen Lock and Tony Smith, Penguin, 1976.

The Ultimate Athlete, George Leonard, Viking (USA), 1975.

Total Fitness, Laurence E. Morehouse and Leonard Gross, Hart-Davis, MacGibbon, 1976.

KIT (article on goggles), Chris Oram, *The Sunday Times*, January 1978.

Effects of ageing upon US masters championship swim performance, Richard H. Rahe and Ransom J. Arthur, *Journal of Sports Medicine and Physical Fitness* (Italy), 1974.

The Fit Athlete, Roy J. Shephard, Oxford University Press, 1978.

Learning to Swim and Dive, Hamilton Smith, Collins, 1973.

Naturally Fit, Bruce Tulloh, Arthur Barker, 1976.

Winning with Wilkie, David Wilkie with Athole Still, Stanley Paul, 1977.

Man's Body, Diagram Group, Corgi, 1977.

Survival Kit, September 1977.

The healthiness of the long-distance runner, Tony Smith, *The Times*, June 1977.

As Easy As Taking A Stroll, James E. Counsilman with Coles Phinizy, *Sports Illustrated*, July 1970.

The Springs of Suffering, Donald Gould, *New Statesman*, October 1977.